During my 48 years as a physiotherapist in my own treatment centers, as well as in some of the large sanitariums including that of Dr. John Harvey Kellogg fame, in Battle Creek, I have had every opportunity to observe the amazing benefits of manual massage. As a means of rehabilitation where physical trauma is involved, it ranks high in the annals of medicine.

The techniques described in Mrs. Carter's book are not something entirely new but have been in use for many years. They neither replace nor substitute for a physician's medical care. However, reflex therapy, often administered by the patient himself through the simple manipulation of prescribed areas of the feet and hands, can amazingly relieve tensions and similar psychosomatic conditions.

The techniques described in Mrs. Carter's book have been developed by experts in the field of reflexology, and we have no hesitation in recommending them to those suffering from the strains and stresses of modern living. For the relief of pain, we know of no other means, short of opiates, to achieve this objective.

CLARENCE R. MUNROE
Registered Technician, Physiotherapy

Mildred Carter has written an outstanding book on foot reflexology which is valuable to the reader on at least three levels:

1. Preventing illness
2. Treating illness in conjunction with other healthcare professionals
3. Helping other people to achieve better health naturally

Foot reflexology has a long history of aiding people in maintaining a healthy body. I first became aware of its value when I was treated by one of my own patients, who was a foot reflexologist. I noticed rapid improvement in my symptoms and began to refer many of my patients to various reflexologists.

Congratulations, Mildred, on all your outstanding books.

Dr. L.E. Dorman, D.O.
Missouri

Healing Yourself
with
FOOT
Reflexology

REVISED & EXPANDED

ALL-NATURAL RELIEF
FOR DOZENS OF AILMENTS

MILDRED CARTER & TAMMY WEBER

Reward Books
a member of Penguin Putnam Inc.
New York

This book is a reference manual based on research by the authors. All techniques and suggestions are to be used at the reader's sole discretion. The opinions expressed herein are not necessarily those of, or endorsed by, the publisher. Information is to be used as a guide to help restore balance within the body, so it can heal itself. The directions stated in this book do not constitute the practice of medicine. Nor are they intended as claims for curing a serious disease and are in no way to be considered as a subsitute for consultation with a duly licensed doctor.

◆ Reward Books
a member of Penguin Putnam Inc.
375 Hudson Street
New York, NY 10014
www.penguinputnam.com

Library of Congress Cataloging-in-Publication Data

Carter, Mildred.
    Healing yourself with foot reflexology / by Mildred Carter and
Tammy Weber.—Rev. and updated ed.
        p.   cm.
    Includes index.
    ISBN 0-7352-0352-0
    1. Healing.   2. Reflexology.   I. Title.
    RM723.R43C374   1996   96-27478
    615.8'22—dc20   CIP

Printed in the United States of America

10   9   8   7   6   5   4   3   2

ACKNOWLEDGMENTS

We gratefully appreciate the emotional support, loving encouragement, and helpful assistance of our loving family and many friends.

A warmhearted recognition goes to our colleagues, Bill Flocco, Elizabeth Fraser, Kevin Kunz, and Jim Ingram for sending us their special scientific reflexology reports and informative journals, thus giving the opportunity to share these positive results with the whole world.

Our gratitude to those who shared their enthusiastic support and special reflexology techniques for the photographs. With fondness we thank: Cynthia Carney, Jennifer Risenhoover, Stephanie Saylors, Brian P. Weber, Kevin Weber, Sandy Weber, and Sherryl D. Weber.

Special credit is due to all of *you* who are giving nature a helping hand by using this natural healing energy to help yourself and others with whom you come in contact. Each life affects another's, and when we can extend a helping hand to show that we care and understand, we are helping to spread the dream of good health throughout this precious universe in which we live. May you, and those you love, always enjoy perfect health.

A WORD FROM THE AUTHORS

From the first time this book was published, in the late 1960s, "reflexology" has come a long way. At that time very few people were familiar with the term, and many had their doubts about its authenticity. Only about 1% of the people we talked to had ever heard of Zone Therapy or Reflex Compression, as it was referred to at that time.

However, it was only a matter of time before *Helping Yourself With Foot Reflexology* became extremely well received. Those who read the book and tried the reflex techniques reported excellent results. Word spread quickly about the amazing drug-free way to natural health called foot reflexology. Today we are happy to report that about 95% of the people we talk to have not only heard the term, but many are using it as an essential part of their life.

We are pleased that individuals everywhere recognize the fact that healing comes from within. Nature has provided the body with an astounding capacity to heal itself; it is up to each one of us to take an active role in learning what the body needs to function properly. Reflexology is not intended as a substitute for medical care. It is a natural process of encouraging the body's own systems to rebalance and self-repair, in the same way as a wound, given time, will heal by itself.

Reflexology can be used by the whole family, from tiny babies to great-grandparents. Working the reflexes, a safe and natural method of improving one's own health, is a privilege each of us can elect to use because we are entitled by birth to keep ourselves free from illness and suffering whenever we can. Young children everywhere can be taught this safe and easy technique, which is nature's plan for perfect health, so they can automatically use it as a natural method of helping themselves, family, and friends throughout their entire lives. Good health is our birthright; reflexology has proven to be a natural-healing breakthrough for thousands of people, and is one means of preventive care that can empower us to govern our own well-being. We must add necessary regimens to our lifestyles to help prevent, or reverse, any troubles that cause pain or discomfort.

Our goal with this book is to reach everyone who wishes to improve physical health and emotional happiness. We hope that this knowledge, presented, as in the past, in a relatively uncomplicated style, will continue to educate those who want to learn the secret for dynamic living, exuberant energy, and youthful vigor.

For this reason this revised book has up-to-date information and new photos, charts, and illustrations. We have substantially expanded the coverage of self-help foot reflexology techniques, and added step-by-step instructions on how to give reflexology to your family and friends.

Reflexology is a wealth of knowledge for people of all ages; this new edition will help you learn how to *listen* to your body, through the tender reflex buttons. Discover how easy it is to help yourself, and others, renew health and harmony the *natural* way.

Wishing you Love and Good Health,
Mildred Carter and Tammy Weber

FOREWORD

It is an honor to introduce this revised edition of Mrs. Carter's seminal work on Foot Reflexology. For nearly three decades the popularity of these treatments has never waned. Worldwide acclaim continues as so many people have seen tremendous suffering relieved through the simple methods outlined in this book.

With the virtual explosion in acceptance of alternative health care, it is the noninvasive therapies that will give us great hope upon entering the 21st century. Reflexology stands with the major contributors in such fields as nutrition, chiropractic, osteopathy, homeopathy and massage.

The human body is at times complex but its needs are ever simple. The body may appreciate the assistance of us well-meaning caregivers but quite prefers minimal interference. This basic tenet is crucial to and shared by many in the alternative care community. Reflexology stands the test of time by adhering to the profound message that the forces present in the building of our bodies are still available for its healing. This therapy makes direct use of these forces by gently removing the blocks to the inherent healing capabilities of the body. By applying pressure to specific areas on the feet, remarkable healing affects are noted in seemingly unconnected and unrelated distant regions.

With the publication of this updated and expanded edition we may now affect even greater healing responses in our patients, our loved ones, and ourselves.

Dr. James Padgett, D.C.
California

WHAT THIS BOOK CAN DO FOR YOU

Your body's health is reflected in your feet. The various organs, nerves, and glands in your body are connected with certain "reflex areas" on the soles, toes, tops, and sides of your feet. This book shows you how possible it is for you, by working these reflex areas in certain simple ways known as "reflexology," to activate natural and prompt relief from practically all your aches and pains. This book also demonstrates, through easy-to-understand reflexology techniques, how to help eliminate practically all types of poor health situations, and often help repair chronic cases that have not yielded completely through other methods of healing.

You can use reflexology to keep yourself, family, and friends in good health by recognizing certain health problems before they may become serious. It is a safe and simple process which promotes better health by reducing stress and tension, strengthening the body's ability to resist attacks of disease, flushing toxins out of the systems, and improving circulation so the body can heal itself. Moreover, reflexing helps achieve protection from health-destroying mental and physical tensions.

This book outlines easy-to-follow self-help methods, as well as directions on how to give another person a reflexology workout. Various skills are described and programmed for specific health situations in simple steps for your use.

Each reflexology technique you apply directly affects the glands, nerves, and organs in your body. The indicated reflexology technique for simple manipulation of these reflex "buttons" on the feet can "signal" an attack, or presence of a malfunction, in a certain part of the body. The recommended reflex technique sends a surge of activity (or stimulating life force) where needed to help clear out congestion, or blockages, and free the flow of energy to restore the body's normal functioning. Helping yourself and others with reflexology requires no expensive equipment or facilities, and is a safe and natural remedy for better health.

This book tells you how to stimulate your reflexes, sharpen your mental abilities, and rejuvenate your circulatory system so that you can look and feel younger. Using foot reflexology will teach you how to be *solely* in charge of your own health.

You can apply reflexology techniques at your convenience at any time and in practically any place. For example, if you wish to take a "reflexology break" for a fast pickup of energy, to recharge your mental vitality, or to find relief from a nagging headache, you can do so at your office or while watching TV at home. You can effectively work the reflexes on yourself or a friend even while on vacation miles away from home. Most often it takes only a few minutes to get beneficial results.

A glance at the index will show the wide range of situations in which reflexology has been used successfully to get significant and concrete benefits. Read the case histories from years of practice with this wonderful healing art to see what it has been able to accomplish. Reflexology is Nature's "push-button" secret for vibrant health, more dynamic living, abundant personal energy, and better living without pain. You can get all these benefits, and even more, by keeping this book within easy reach for reference when confronted with a perplexing health situation.

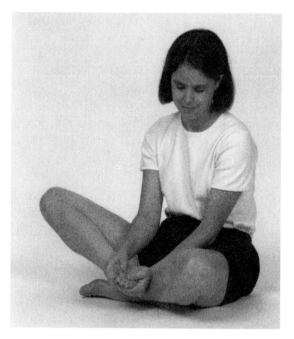

Photo 1.   Dissolve stress and tension with reflexology. It is the key to complete relaxation.

INTRODUCTION

This book, divided into three parts for your convenience, will show you how much fun and how easy it is to achieve and maintain vibrant health for yourself and for those you care about. Each section includes comprehensive photos and illustrations to show graphically various reflex areas, techniques, and positions. These time-tested methods are extremely effective to relax and regenerate the whole body.

PART ONE: LEARNING THE BASICS OF REFLEXOLOGY.

Here we describe the theory, principles, and benefits of this wonderful healing art. By studying the diagrams and techniques, you will become acquainted with the reflexes in the feet and how they correspond to the glands, organs, and total body structure. Charts will help you visualize the zones and divisions of the body. You will learn the grammar of reflexology to help yourself, family, and friends regain better health and well-being through this special language of "reflex signals."

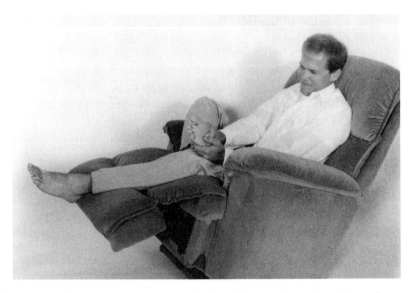

Photo 2. For best results, use a comfortable position when doing foot reflexology.

PART TWO: THE STUDY OF HOW YOU CAN HELP YOUR-SELF WITH FOOT REFLEXOLOGY.

Whether you need basic relaxation from a stress-filled day, or are convalescing after an illness, you can use the simple method of reflexology on yourself. No one knows your body as well as you do; it is completely natural to work your own reflexes, just as you instinctively rub sore muscles when they are stiff to make them feel better. Thus does nature encourage self-stimulation.

You will learn many special reflex techniques that will help you to relax, as well as stimulate circulation for an improved blood supply beneficial in combating particular ailments. Find out the importance of each reflex, and how miraculously nature has linked each one to a corresponding body part. Illustrations at the beginning of each chapter show where the gland or organ is located in the body and where the reflex can be found in the feet. Give yourself time to learn the pressure points and how they relate with your body; then you can proceed effectively to feel restored and full of renewed vitality.

PART THREE: HOW TO EASILY HELP YOUR FAMILY AND FRIENDS WITH REFLEXOLOGY.

This section will instruct you on how to help others normalize and balance their bodies. As you learn these special skills to help others, you will also notice the unfolding of a new inner sense of compassion. Take all the time you need to study and properly learn the art of reflexology. When you develop a feeling for this healing energy, you will be giving more than comfort, warmth, and pleasure to someone you care about. You will also be giving that person reassurance for renewed vitality and wellness. Reflexology is wonderful to use on one's self, but like love, it is best when given to another.

Mildred Carter and Tammy Weber

Table of Contents

How to Improve Life with Reflexology

CHAPTER 1

How Reflexology Works

Reflexology is a scientific technique of applying pressure to reflexes that have a definite effect on the normal functioning of all parts of the body. Properly performed, this reflex work sends stimuli to various organs, glands, and nerves in the body. Tenderness at particular points, which are most commonly found in the feet and hands, may indicate congestion within the body. The purpose of reflexology is to promote balance and normalization, to reduce tension, to revitalize, reactivate, regenerate, heal, and bring the whole system into harmony and a state of good health, *naturally.*

Its simplicity can be disarming but there can be no question of its effectiveness in restoring health and vitality to individuals of any age. It uses no drugs or salves and only a minimum of equipment.

The study of foot reflexology will help you understand and activate the body's vital life force. The entire body is reflected on the feet through a system of reflexes. Application of pressure to reflex points promotes vital energy that runs vertically through the body (the right foot corresponds to the right side of the body, the left foot to the left side).

Pain, discomfort, and many diseases anywhere in the body may be eliminated by working the reflexes in the corresponding zones of the feet. Keep in mind that you do not work the area of pain itself;

3

the reflex "button," though far removed from the ailing organ, will perform this miracle for you.

A BRIEF HISTORY

Reflexology originated several thousand years B.C. Its roots have been traced back to Africa, China, Egypt, India, Japan, and Russia. Variations of this ancient healing art are illustrated in ancient books and journals; even pictographs over 2,330 years old have been found showing Egyptians working on feet and hands to promote good health.

Reflexology was rediscovered in the United States by the American physician, the late Dr. William H. Fitzgerald. A respected graduate of the University of Vermont, he worked at Boston City Hospital and Central London Nose and Throat Hospital. He spent time working in Vienna, and then returned to St. Francis Hospital in Hartford, Connecticut as senior nose and throat surgeon. He was an active member of most of the American medical societies, and brought his discovery to the attention of the medical profession in 1913. At that time the term used was "zone therapy."

He divided the body into ten longitudinal zones of energy, five on each side, each extending from the tips of the toes, and tips of fingers, to corresponding zones of the head. Dr. Fitzgerald observed that by applying direct pressure to certain areas of the body with his hands or with a small tool, he could "stop pain," or produce an anesthetic reaction in a corresponding part of the body within that same zone. Fitzgerald and colleagues Dr. Edwin Bowers and Dr. George Starr White, of Los Angeles, California, further popularized zone therapy by crusading its merits to practitioners and laymen alike.

The late Eunice D. Ingham blazed a path to this unique way to health through her many years of work and association with Dr. Joe Shelby Riley, his wife, and other practicing physicians, by whom the foundation theory of this work was set forth. Their contribution to this natural healing process and regeneration of the body through working the reflexes in the feet is an invaluable part of its history.

It was my good fortune to have studied under Eunice Ingham. I will always be grateful to her for enabling me to bring relief to so many suffering people and to see their joy in regaining health and vitality when all hope had been seemingly lost. Now I give you this simple, unique, but scientific method of bringing the same results into your own life.

HEALING FORCES RELEASED THROUGH REFLEXOLOGY

What will reflexology do for you? This book will show you by pictures and charts a simple method of how to stimulate these reflexes to bring relief of pains and diseases.

Not only will you learn how to distinguish and cope with many illnesses, aches, and pains, but also you will discover how to use the healing forces of nature to bring relief, and in many cases complete healing, by the simple technique of "working" the reflexes.

You will use the healing forces of nature to restore glandular vitality, beauty, and health. "The fountain of youth is within you."

You can get almost immediate relief from many aches and pains by pressing a certain reflex button under the skin of your foot or hand, and "working" it for a few moments in a certain way.

Many headaches will vanish almost immediately by manipulating the big toes, as they contain the reflexes to the head.

I have seen hands and feet, badly twisted by painful arthritis, straightened back to normal as a result of properly working the reflexes which relaxed the body and returned it to its balanced acidity level.

Reflexology can send nature's healing forces to help a failing heart.

It can stop the pain of hemorrhoids almost immediately.

It can halt a sore throat in minimal time.

You will be able to slow the advance of old age and senility. By the correct use of reflexology you can reactivate the body's natural processes of rejuvenation and regeneration of cells, and bring new life to those who are already senile.

You will relax the nervous tension of your body and be able to sleep better. You will be able to relieve others of pain and illness, through the blessed use of reflexology.

You will be able to improve circulation flow and impede delivery of oxygen to the cells. Properly working the reflexes will help the body *balance itself naturally.*

You will learn the relationship of glands, and the influence they have on your health, your mentality, your life.

Reflexology can be an important step in your journey to health. As your reflex-work progresses, each pressure point is another step along the path to good health.

How does this work?

Reflexology requires no medicinal pills or shots, no special programmed diet (except where this might be otherwise indicated), and no elaborate equipment; moreover, the techniques may be applied to people of all ages. Healing forces are released by movements of energy that travel through the body to balance and energize. This vital energy promotes improved health by reducing tension and pain, as well as by escalating the strength of the body's functions. Reflexing is one of the quickest and most natural ways known to relieve distress and restore energy and good health, without negative side effects.

Reflexology will free you from sickness and suffering, and fear of pain, *when used correctly.*

As you gain a deeper understanding of how powerful reflexology is, you will appreciate how it contributes to your wellness, how it balances the overall functioning of the body, and how it enhances the body's remarkable ability to repair itself! You will learn the power of thoughts concerning your health, beauty, and happiness. To be happy is to be healthy and beautiful. Sadness, anger, and fear create tension, which results in sickness and rapid aging. Reflexology relaxes tension!

Once you understand these initial steps, you will learn how to use reflexology to benefit yourself and all mankind. This book will open the door to a different, scientific way to health, vitality, and the joy of living. The information, charts, and photos will act as your guide, and will help you to understand how safe and effective reflexology is, and how you can give nature a helping hand by using this natural healing energy.

Step-by-Step Guide to the Foot/Body Relationship

As you study the following reflexology charts, you will become acquainted with the positions of the reflexes in the feet and their corresponding relationship to the vital parts of the body. All diagrams graphically shown in the feet represent *reflex areas.*

EXPLANATION OF CHARTS A AND B

Look closely at Charts A and B. Notice how the right foot corresponds to the right side of the body; the left foot corresponds to the left side of the body. If you get a clear picture of this in your mind, then it will be easier for you to find the reflexes in your feet.

It will become natural for you to know the position of each reflex and its corresponding part in the body, after you have practiced working the reflexes a few times.

Notice how the head corresponds with the big toe. Look at Chart A and find the position of the pituitary gland in the head. Now look at Chart B and find the reflex to the pituitary gland, in the center of the big toe. The pituitary gland in the head will be stimulated by working the corresponding reflex in the toe. Since the location of this gland is in the center of the head, you will work the reflex in both the right and the left toes. (Explanation of Charts A and B continued on page 13)

7

VISUAL GUIDE TO THE INNER STRUCTURE OF THE BODY

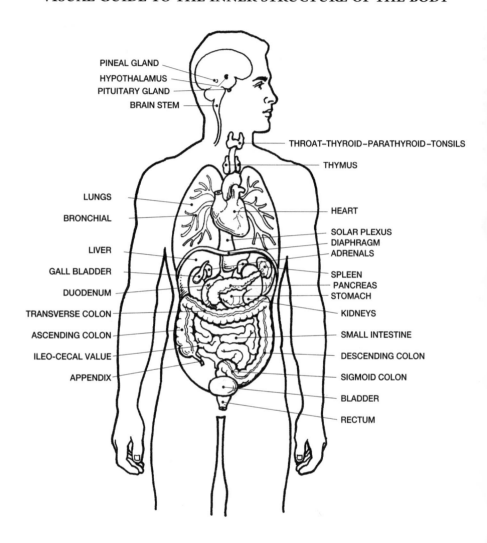

PINEAL GLAND
HYPOTHALAMUS
PITUITARY GLAND
BRAIN STEM

THROAT–THYROID–PARATHYROID–TONSILS
THYMUS

LUNGS
BRONCHIAL

HEART

SOLAR PLEXUS
DIAPHRAGM
LIVER
ADRENALS

GALL BLADDER
SPLEEN
PANCREAS
DUODENUM
STOMACH

TRANSVERSE COLON
KIDNEYS

ASCENDING COLON
SMALL INTESTINE

ILEO-CECAL VALUE
DESCENDING COLON

APPENDIX
SIGMOID COLON

BLADDER

RECTUM

Right Side   **Left Side**

Chart A. The human body has many parts; many overlap each other so it is hard to place them all in their anatomical order. Someone looking for a specific gland or organ can visualize where it is placed in the body, and get a general idea of the other major organs that are located nearby. Look for the Guide-at-a-glance drawings throughout the book to help you better visualize the interior areas of the body.

FOOT REFLEXOLOGY CHART

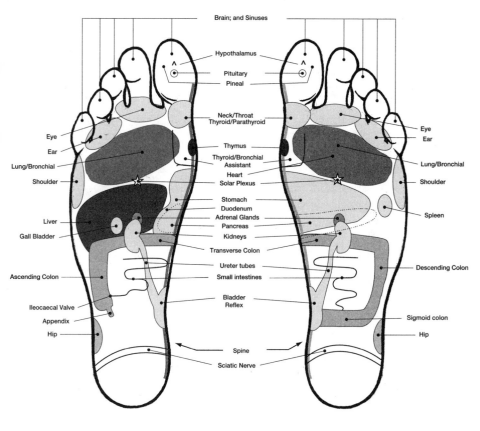

Sole of Right Foot   Sole of Left Foot

Chart B. The feet represent small mirrors, which reflect an image of the whole body. Compare Chart A with Chart B and you will notice a reflection of internal organs and glands on the soles of the feet. These charts will help you visualize how the feet are like miniature maps of the body. Tender reflex points in the feet represent trouble within the corresponding organism. Specific reflex pressure to the tender areas helps improve circulation, encourages various systems to flush out toxins, and helps permeate every living cell with renewed vital energy which promotes the body to heal itself.

SIDE VIEW OF FEET

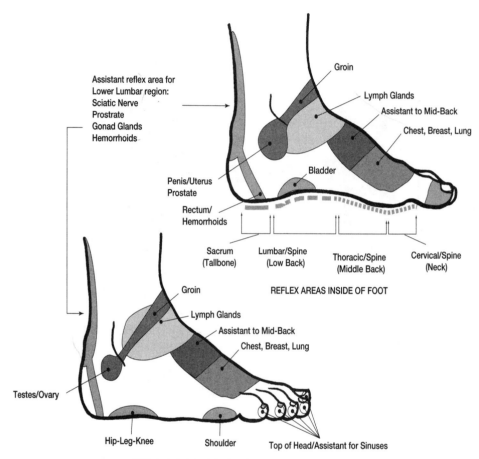

Assistant reflex area for
Lower Lumbar region:
Sciatic Nerve
Prostrate
Gonad Glands
Hemorrhoids

Groin

Lymph Glands
Assistant to Mid-Back
Chest, Breast, Lung

Penis/Uterus
Prostate

Bladder

Rectum/
Hemorrhoids

Sacrum   Lumbar/Spine
(Tallbone)   (Low Back)   Thoracic/Spine   Cervical/Spine
                                     (Middle Back)   (Neck)

Groin   REFLEX AREAS INSIDE OF FOOT

Lymph Glands
Assistant to Mid-Back
Chest, Breast, Lung

Testes/Ovary

Hip-Leg-Knee   Shoulder   Top of Head/Assistant for Sinuses

REFLEX AREAS OUTSIDE OF FOOT

Chart C. Reflex areas that are located on the inside and outside of the feet. Notice that the gonad (sex gland) reflexes are not on the bottoms of the feet like the reflexes to most of the organs of the body but are protected up on the sides. These glands are very important to good health, and should be reflexed a few minutes whenever you work on the feet. The cord up the back of the leg contains assistant reflexes to the lower region of the body. Only one reflex to this area is neccessary per session.

TOP VIEW OF FEET

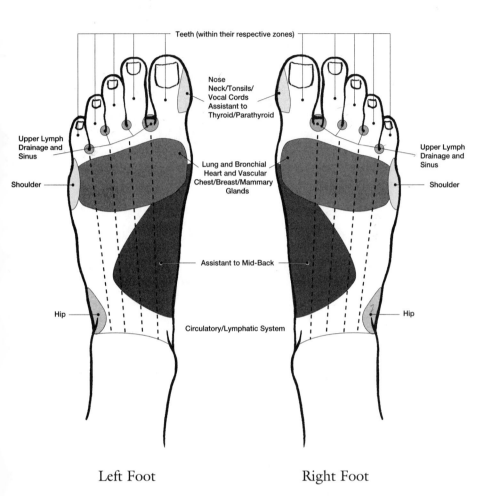

Left Foot   Right Foot

Chart D. By reflexing the tops of the feet, you will fine-tune these basic reflex areas that correspond to the front of the body.

When giving reflexology to another person, turn this chart upside down for a visual understanding of the feet.

THE ENDOCRINE SYSTEM AND ITS REFLEXES

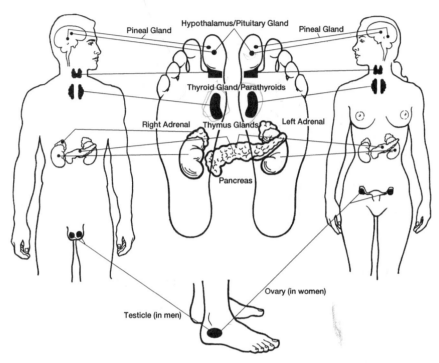

*Highlighting the Endocrine Glands Activities

Hypothalamus regulates chemical production.
Pituitary controls other endocrine glands.
Pineal is the pituitary helper.
Thyroid controls emotional stability.
Parathyroid helps the thyroid keep the body balanced.
Thymus guards against infection and gives energy.
Pancreas secrets insulin and controls blood sugar.
Adrenal produces adrenaline for energy, helps promote desires and courage.
Gonads responsible for personality and drive.

Notice how nature designed the arrangement of these glands, mostly lined up in the center of the head and body.

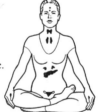

*For additional information of these specialized glands see Chapter 25.

Chart E. The all-important endocrine system controls the body's functions and rhythms, by secreting a variety of chemicals called hormones, into your bloodstream. The hypothalamus controls hormone production. The pituitary "Master" gland produces hormones, and stimulates the various other glands to generate their own hormones, which in turn are carried off to varying cells in the body.

The neck and throat correspond with the base of the large toe where it is fastened onto the foot.

Notice that the eye and ear reflexes are just below the smaller toes. Since we have an eye and ear on each side of the head, there will be reflexes on the same side of each foot. The body has two lungs, one on each side. On the chart you see the reflexes to the lungs in a matching area on the left and right foot.

As we progress down the body we will see how the spine corresponds with the bones along the inside of the foot, from the mid joint of the big toe down to the heel bone. At the end of the spine in the body we likewise come to the end of the bony structure in the foot. If there is pain in the center of the back, you would work the center of this bony structure in the foot (see the positions on the chart). If there is a centralized pain of the spine, you will not have any difficulty finding the right location of the reflex to it on the foot, as you will find it very tender when you press on it.

Notice how the liver is on the right side of the body and the reflexes to the liver are on the right foot, in a somewhat similar position.

We see the appendix is located on the right side of the body at the beginning of the colon; the corresponding reflex to the appendix is on the right foot at the beginning of the colon reflex.

You should now comprehend how the position of the reflexes in the feet corresponds to the location of the organs and glands of the body.

THE BODY'S ENERGY ZONES

Every body has natural energy channels, also referred to as the life force, or the essence of life, chi, prana, or the divine spark of internal energy. Other languages may refer to it by another name. Whether the term is familiar or not, we must all realize the obvious presence of this "life energy" by its strength and effectiveness.

Nature and the Divine Energy

This world is one of life, energy, and strength, all of which are Nature's wonders. The body has a remarkable ability to regenerate itself, and is a wondrous conductor of Nature's energies . . . energies with the strength to renew our physical and mental health. Most sickness is caused by an obstruction of a physical or energetic nature, such as fat, mucus, or poor energy flow. This blockage within the body hinders circulation and interferes with the normal activity of the organs, nerves, and muscles. When you remove the obstruction, circulation of energy returns and balance is maintained; then healing can take place naturally.

The Zone Theory

The zone theory holds that there are ten energy channels, "zones" that run longitudinally through the body and along which the vital life force (energy) travels. Applying pressure to the reflexes at the base of these zones stimulates a subtle force of nature's healing energy which cleans away obstructions, thereby promoting a renewed energy flow. This contributes to a more efficient functioning of the body systems.

This subtle energy force also helps bring about both improved circulation and the return of the body to a healthy balance. It is significantly important in reducing stress and encourages deep relaxation.

EXPLANATION OF CHART F

Energy zones are not visible, yet by looking at Chart F, you will be able to imagine how these channels of energy run lengthwise up the body from the feet (and hands) to the head. Pressure to reflexes stimulates healing energy to various sections of the body.

There are ten longitudinal zones, five on each side of the body, one zone for each toe (and for each finger).

- Zone One . . . originates in each big toe (and each thumb) and runs up the center of the body, to the centerline in the head.
- Zone Two . . . runs alongside zone one on both the right and left sides of the body, up to the top of the head.
- Zone Three . . . travels up the middle toes (and middle fingers) on the right and left sides of the body, to the top of the head.

TEN ENERGY ZONES

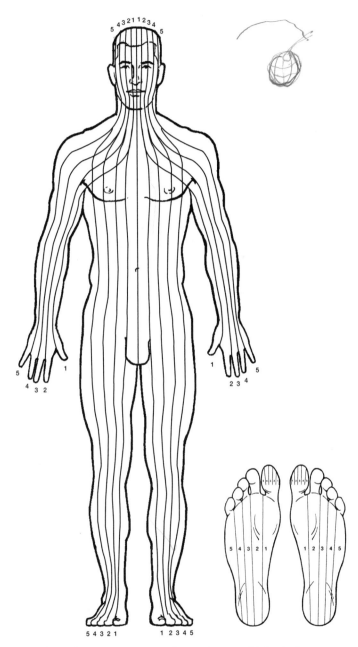

Chart F. Each numbered zone represents the pathway which vital energy flows. Pressure applied to a sore reflex will indicate tension or imbalance within that same zone (or zones) of the body.

- Zone Four . . . is in the fourth toes (and fingers) on both sides of the body, and moves up through the body to the top of the head.
- Zone Five . . . runs up the little toes (and fingers) and makes its journey up the extreme outside of the body, to the outer sides of the head.

"There are ten invisible electrical currents through the body . . . they are in line with the toes and fingers."

—Dr. William Fitzgerald

After studying these charts, you can understand how working the reflex areas in the feet will stimulate the whole body. You will not be treating just one congested area; you will be sending an invigorating, life-giving flow of circulation to every part of the body.

DIVISIONS OF THE BODY AND FEET

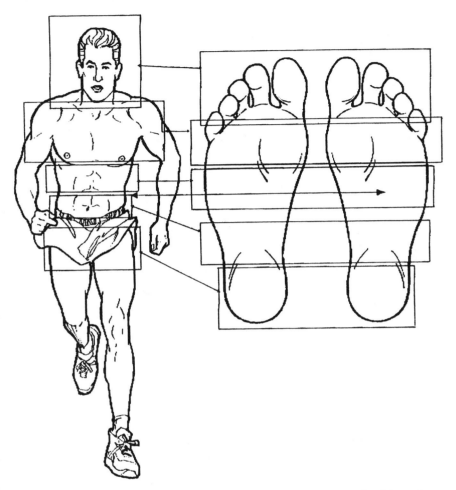

Chart G. Look at this chart for a fuller understanding of the body's regions and how they correspond to the divisions on the feet.

(1) • Press the reflexes in the toes to activate brain and other parts of the head.

(2) • Reflexes in the balls of feet (and top of feet) relate to the chest area.

(3) • Across the center of feet is the "Waistline" which matches up with the center of body.

(4) • Lower region of feet conform to the body's lower torso.

(5) • Reflexes in the heels and ankles coincide with the pelvic region.

The Benefits of Reflexology

There is an ancient Arabian proverb which says, "He who has health, has hope; and he who has hope, has everything."

Probably no one would agree to this as readily and enthusiastically as the person who is or has been ill, for usually one must know sickness before one is able to appreciate a sound body.

If retaining or regaining health were a single process linked to one line of endeavor or one specific habit, pursuing it would be simple. But a full, abundant life involves so many factors that every person should be constantly alert to ways to get the most out of his or her years on earth.

God not only created a marvelous human body, but also placed the resources needed upon the earth so both men and women could remain healthy and happy.

ELECTRICAL NATURE OF REFLEXES

The electrical reflexes in the bottoms of the feet and in the palms of the hands which correspond to every part of the human body represent one of the most miraculous means given to man, and probably one of the least familiar.

These were placed there in the beginning when man was made to go naked, walking on his bare feet over rugged terrain.

Early man roamed over plains and through forests. He stepped on objects which pressed into his feet, reaching the tiny electrical reflexes and furnishing a natural massage. This natural form of stimulation broke and loosened any small crystals that might have formed there in the nerve structures or blood vessels, causing congestion, which would, in turn, slow the flow of blood to the part of the body corresponding to the reflex involved. The electrical shock stimulated the portion of the body to which that part of the foot corresponded, and the body as a whole was in rhythm with the universe.

Why Early Man Was Healthier

Early man was healthy because of this natural reflex pressure during his daily activities. When blood is slowed in any place by an obstruction, that place or organ becomes sluggish, just as a pond becomes stagnant when running water no longer flows through it.

Today we have footwear. We have sidewalks. We have smooth, soft, green lawns. Consequently, this natural stimulation of old *is no more*. But this does not mean that modern man must forego its benefits.

He is quite capable of managing this stimulation, either manually or by use of a "Deluxe-Foot-Roller" which comes complete with a book of diagrams and explicit directions. (See back of book for details.)

I have had so many personal experiences of over the years with family, friends, and clients that I have relieved through reflexology that I find myself wanting to tell all of them at once. Reflexology is so simple and natural that it is safe to use on anyone from the youngest baby to the eldest person. And its benefits? They are positive!

Husband Struck with Heart Attack

As is so often the case, tragedy brought about my original interest in the matter of achieving good health. My husband was struck down with a heart attack when he was only 34. There had been no warning, at least not one which we recognized, and the doctors at that time appeared to know little about his trouble.

He was put to bed for a year. There I was with two school-age children and a baby only two months old.

I always wanted to know the "why" of everything; this situation of my husband's illness was no exception.

There were bound to be reasons, cures, even preventatives. Begging the doctors for information would get me nowhere for I already realized they were in a quandary. What I sought was the *real* answer, the simple method Nature had given us in the beginning.

So rewarding and fascinating was the knowledge gradually acquired that I never became discouraged, searching always, learning, applying them for my husband.

Through proper diet and mild exercise, he slowly overcame his bad heart and lived for many years.

How Author Reclaimed Youthfulness

By the time I was in my middle 40's, I realized that my youthful face was showing fine lines. My skin was a bit flabby. I did not feel the usual lightness in my body, and again I undertook to meet this challenge of oncoming old age. I began a system of exercise and was quite satisfied with the results until one day I met a woman from Arizona, who told me of this system of reflex compression on feet and palms. She gave me a treatment, and I was amazed at how good I felt when she was finished. Not only was I revitalized, but my feet felt as though I walked on a cushion of air.

At first I did not understand that this pressure therapy could be added to the knowledge I already had rather than being a thing apart, so I gave much thought to whether or not I should pursue it in place of exercise, diet, and the other programs I had acquired through the years.

I felt I had found the answer about foot reflex therapy when I remembered all the passages in the Bible which had to do with the anointing of the feet.

A Reflex-a-Day Helps Keep Pain Away

The practice of *reflexology* is one of Nature's ways to better health and well-being. It stimulates energy to sick glands, and enables them to

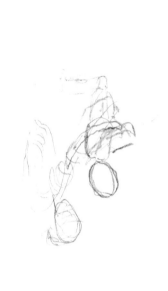

return to a healthy state. The applications of reflexology are limitless—here are a few case histories.

Kidneys, Ovaries, and Hemorrhoids Healed

A friend had suffered for years with a kidney ailment and a diseased ovary so that she was almost physically disabled. Three treatments relieved her of her symptoms, and when the course was finished, she also admitted to troublesome hemorrhoids which no longer plagued her (which was an extra bonus of the reflex sessions).

Epileptic Seizures

A woman brought her son to me, telling me he had been subject to epileptic seizures since he was nine years old. He was then having as many as 27 spells a night at the age of 24.

The tender spots in his feet were many, denoting the condition of the main glands. This profusion made it difficult to decide which glands were causing his seizures. However, one immediate treatment lessened his spells to one that night.

A few more reflex sessions enabled him to discard most of his medication and he experienced an average of one seizure a week. The tenderness had left the bottoms of his feet and his foot sessions were reduced from every other day to one a week.

One sore spot remained which was located up under the big toe, a reflex to the parathyroid gland. "The doctors believe that is the root of his trouble," his mother declared, "but they could only give him medicine for it." Nevertheless, he had found the road to recovery.

From Heart Weakness to Rejuvenation

In the earlier years of my giving reflexology, a woman in her late 60's was brought to me. She had been in bed for three months, her heart presumably bad. She was helped up the steps and was breathing with difficulty. Her trembling hands denoted how nervous she was.

At that time, I had little experience in handling a heart patient and I undertook it with considerable care.

But I need not have been overly concerned, for my patient grew calm. She no longer panted. Her hands lay calmly in her lap.

She came to me every other day for a week, at the end of which time she was in good spirits, walking spryly up the steps without help.

Her sessions lessened to one a week, and as I worked on her feet, she would tell me of the miraculous changes throughout her body. The woman was actually going through a period of rejuvenation. Her sense of smell had been dulled and now she was able to gather in odors. Her sense of taste had been practically gone and now she enjoyed her food again.

The woman began to walk in her garden; then she was able to take the bus downtown shopping.

I found myself warning her, for the heart, being a muscle, had to have time to build back its strength. It was weak from not doing its proper share of work.

Some four years thereafter, I chanced to meet the woman's daughter and inquired about my former patient.

"Mother goes all around the country by bus, visiting relatives, having a delightful time," she told me.

Reflexology Benefits for Older People

Foot reflexology is especially good for elderly people, for it rejuvenates the entire body, giving new life to the glands and cells. Blood flow slows over the years. Naturally, glands and cells become sluggish. Stimulating a new flow of blood to these tired places brings new life, clears glands and cells of accumulated poisons, and reestablishes harmony and balance among body functions.

Cataracts of the Eyes

To an elderly woman with cataracts I could not promise any encouragement that reflexology would give her any relief, but she insisted that I try. Her husband brought her 200 miles once a week to see me. Before she had made many such journeys, her near-blindness had been relieved sufficiently so that she could read the advertisements on the signboards enroute. She no longer needed to be led into my office, and she was able to see the denomination of the paper money she handled.

A Puzzling Illness Solved

An acquaintance was troubled with female disorders, and although she was only in her 30's her doctor had arranged for her to have a hysterectomy. The doctor was primarily a surgeon, and I urged this woman to seek another opinion before she submitted to surgery.

She visited a doctor in an adjacent town, one specializing in female disorders; he declared she needed only minor surgery, so slight it could be taken care of in a doctor's office. But he also suggested one more examination for yet another opinion.

The third doctor said she had ulcers and put her on an ulcer diet. About a month later, she called me and said she was very sick.

When I reached her home, I was alarmed. The woman had pulled off all her clothing. She lay on the couch gasping and writhing. I quickly started to work on her foot, and she soon began to grow more quiet.

Finally I was able to talk with her. She said she kept having these spells and was so terribly sick she was sure she was dying.

I had been home no longer than ten minutes when she summoned me to return. The second treatment again brought relief. When I reached home after this second trip, I consulted with my own doctor. I did not want to get involved with a serious heart condition, although there was no indication of it in the reflexes of her feet. He said he would make a house call and check.

The woman's heart was perfect. She had no high blood pressure. "I have no idea what is causing these spells," he declared. "Perhaps if she had been having one when I was there . . ."

He reasoned that the only cause of such pain would be from an ulcer healing, if it were an exceedingly large one.

"You are coming home with me," I told her, and so I gathered her up along with her children and took them to my house. We had not been there more than a few minutes when she moaned that another attack was coming on.

Immediately I got busy on her feet, and by now I believed I knew the seat of her troubles. She needed something done for the liver and gallbladder. I worked the reflexes governing these organs and was rewarded with a deep sigh. She closed her eyes and mur-

mured weakly, "It is as if a huge blanket of pain has been lifted from me."

"You go to my doctor tomorrow," I suggested, "and tell him you believe your trouble is in the region of your liver and gallbladder. Avoid telling him why you believe this."

He sent her to the hospital for tests and x-rays, which corroborated my opinion. The woman had gallstones, and surgery removed 13 of good size.

My doctor, aware of my work, has never tried to interfere. In fact, another doctor in a neighboring town has often sent for a woman who was a reflexologist to solve puzzling cases which he could not diagnose.

Reflexology for Pets

My story of reflexology and its individual cases would be less than complete were I to omit the story of Inky, our three-year-old Pomeranian dog. This is a breed subject to asthma attacks. Inky had an alarming attack one Sunday when we had guests. I kept rubbing his throat, giving him something to inhale to aid him in his breathing.

His difficulties did not lessen after we retired; he was in such discomfort that the family was kept awake by his attempts to breathe. Finally, I brought him to my side of the bed, rolled him over on his back, and began to rub his feet.

Certainly I had not the slightest notion where to rub a dog's foot to ease him of his asthma. But with great care I worked each pad of each toe, then the center large pad.

After five minutes his panic-stricken struggle to breathe eased. I discovered the small extra toe high up on the foot was the most tender spot.

All four feet thus treated, he relaxed and I fell asleep. I was awakened later in the night by his wheezing, but this time it was not as loud. When I called him to the bed from his own blanket in the room, he came readily, lying on his back, feet upturned for a second treatment!

Almost at once his breathing became easier and when I drifted off to sleep the second time, my little dog patient was slumbering also.

For all the rest of the years our pet was with us, he had few asthma attacks; when he did, reflexology quickly relieved him.

HAND AND BODY REFLEXES

The healing power of reflexology is Nature's way to perfect health. When using this method you are the facilitator for Nature, stimulating the divine energy that helps speed up the healing forces throughout the body. Proper application of pressure to various reflex areas on the hands, feet or body promotes renewed balance and normal functioning in all systems, naturally.

Hand Reflexes

The position of the reflexes found in the hand are basically the same as those found in the foot, and on the same side of the body. However, because of the difference in size and shape of the hand, you will need to refer to a "hand reflex chart" to make sure of the correct reflex locations. Since hands are more exposed and do such a great amount of work, these reflexes are a bit less sensitive than those in the feet.

The tender palm reflexes of an active person are generally worked out in the day's usual routine. This is nature's way of stimulating the body's circulation. However, if an individual becomes inactive, never using the hands and fingers to grip with or pick up objects, the buttons under the skin of the palms *must be reflexed* to promote renewed circulation. The thumb and fingers of the opposite hand can work these reflexes for renewed stimulation, but if the thumb or fingers are weak, sore or disabled, a self-help tool such as the "Reflex Probe" or the "Reflex Massager" will be especially efficient in searching for tender buttons.

Body Reflexes

Doctors Fitzgerald, White, and Bowers, all MDs, and Dr. R. Wilborn, DC, were among the physicians who believed their mission was to teach as well as to heal. They were all concerned with *prevention* and the *cure of disease*. These doctors helped many people stay healthy with body reflexology, or "zone therapy" as it was referred to in the early 1900s. They taught how simple it was to use *direct pressure on a certain reflex area* of the body, head, tongue, hands, or feet to get an *anesthetic* effect in a far removed area within the same zone.

They divided the head and the whole body, even the tongue, longitudinally into ten zones, five on each side of a median line. Both hands and feet had five zones each.

The doctors proved that it was possible to anesthetize certain body parts, from head throughout the extremities, by pressure to a particular reflex point on yet another part of the body within individual zones, or groups of zones.

Dr. Fitzgerald and his colleagues used another method of body-reflex-work, which was known at that time as "hooking-work," or "pressure-work." We now call this technique "working the 'referral areas.'" For example, if there was pain in the *left shoulder*, and moving or pressing around it caused discomfort, then you could "refer" your reflex-work to a corresponding part of the body, in this case, the *left hip*. (This would be the same on the right shoulder, of course, to work on the right hip, etc.).

Whether you need a boost of energy in the morning, or to unwind after a stress-filled day, your hands, feet, and body can be a great benefit to you. They are always with you and at your convenience, you can work the reflexes in a moment's notice. Reflexology is a fast, effective, and convenient way to preserve health and renew your well-being.

How a Sister Helps Her Brother with Reflexology

My Special Client, by S.B.

All of the people I give reflexology to are special, but this is my brother and I asked his permission to write this story and he said I could. My brother Bob has cerebral palsy from a birth accident, asthma, and many other health problems. He has had a very rough life. First learning to walk around age of five with leg braces, surgery after surgery. Then he did learn to walk on his own but his motor skills are not normal.

I asked my brother if I could practice reflexology on him and he said yes. So he started coming over twice a week. I did his hands and feet. The motor skills were so bad in his hands he could only bring his thumb to the bottom of the knuckle of his hands. I continued working on his hands and feet. I noticed an improvement in his motor skills.

Then I started working up pressure points in his arm around the elbow and up to the shoulder, down the sides of the spinal column, and over the hip sockets. Then I worked his legs, did pressure points up the legs around the knee, up to the groin.

A miracle did happen! By the thirteenth session, for the first time in his life, he had mobility in his hands and he could bring his thumb to the top finger pads! His speech improved and one night, while I was working on him, he said, "Don't make me too healthy now, I'm not used to this." I just chuckled. He could not believe the improvement himself, watching this happen through reflexology. He is doing great, thanks to your books, course, and one of your graduate students, for helping me learn reflexology. Bob said when I write this I am supposed to say "thank you" from him also.

Maybe other people with cerebral palsy would benefit from reflexology like Bob has. It is a great feeling for me, that my goals and dreams are becoming a reality.

Love,
S.B., Wisconsin

EUROPEAN METHODS VS. REFLEXOLOGY

In Germany, there is a method of treatment being used by two doctors who claim extraordinary success.

Doctor Ferdinand Huneke and his brother, Walter, use a healing method which is called *neural therapy*. They inject a local anesthetic in certain parts of the body to bring about instant healing.

A health magazine article stated that the method of achieving this instant healing effect was through the nervous system, specifically through the vegetative (autonomic) nervous system. Neural therapy deals with an unspecific stimulus type of treatment. A directed stimulus put into the right place is capable of inducing real healing through a lightning-quick change of the electrophysical state of the vegetative nerves, with accompanying instant freedom from pain and discomfort.

With neural therapy, doctors have to study the case history of the patient in order to find the pathological connections which induce healing. They study all previous illnesses since this might be an old injury that left scars, an infection that was still present in a different part of the body.

It is claimed that the exhaustive searching back into a patient's past medical history opens up many questions for researchers in the field.

A neural therapist who has to observe and ask questions needs great empathy with the patient, who is not able to understand why an old, forgotten injury or sickness could, after many years, be responsible for a quite different illness.

Only an extensive case history makes the discovery of a connection possible in *neural therapy.* In reflexology, we do not have to know about past injuries or illnesses. *They will show up in the tenderness of the reflexes in the bottoms of the feet if they are still affecting the patient's health.*

Reflex therapy is similar to neural therapy in that instantaneous healing is not unknown in either of these two forms of treatment. This is so probably because the same electrophysical processes are employed in both therapies, although in a different and simpler way in reflexology.

Sometimes, after certain damages, the body is unable to recuperate completely and regain its former condition. A permanent change remains in the tissues, and often this goes unrecognized. This is reflected in the electrophysical relationship of the tissues. A field of disturbance is thus created, from which faulty stimuli may be directed to any other part of the body or organism by the electrically structured vegetative nerves. It is very possible that any chronic disease may be triggered by a field of disturbance that can be in any part of the organism.

Scars as a Source of Body Disturbance

Scars, in particular, have proven to be a field of disturbance for a great number of disorders.

This brings us back to reflexology! When treating all the specific reflexes on the feet, electrical energy runs up to every part of the body. If there is trouble from an old scar or illness, the pressure point which corresponds to this complication is reached; thus the healing powers of the body are activated.

It may be surprising to realize that an old scar on your leg could be causing the pain in your head! It is also equally gratifying to know that you have only to do a thorough job of foot reflexology and the rest will take care of itself.

REFLEXOLOGY IS OFTEN USED WITH CONVENTIONAL MEDICAL CARE

Keep in mind that the techniques of reflexology do not contradict traditional medical practice. Many doctors, chiropractors, and physical therapists are using it along with conventional medical care in various hospitals and health care clinics.

Indeed, because of research and study, reflexology is now being accepted around the world by increasing numbers of physicians who recognize its benefits and recommend it as a means of preventative health care. *Health Wise News* reports that Dr. Bruce Blenenstock, head of the Department of Psychiatry and Behavioral Medicine at the Palo Alto Medical Foundation, says, "Only a fool would discount healing systems that have been adopted around the world and maintained for thousands of years. And those systems often refer to an energy, a 'life force,' or spiritual element that must be considered an integral part of health."

Research Reports

The Spring, 1996 issue of *Reflexions,* printed an article titled "Reflexology Research Around the World" by Kevin and Barbara Kunz. Reflexology is being studied at Columbia University, and is taught by noted cardiothoracic surgeon Dr. Mehmet Oz to his medical students. Seen on the *ABC Nightly News* January 11, 1996 "American Agenda, with Peter Jennings," Dr. Oz tells his medical students, "We have a charge as an academic institution to study these things" (referring to natural alternative therapies); moreover, he has convinced other doctors and hospital officials to allow him to use the work of alternative practitioners with his cardiovascular patients.

Also the Kunz reflexology journal, *Reflexions,* reprinted a *New York Times* article which refers to Dr. Oz as "probably the most accomplished 35-year-old cardiothoracic surgeon in the country" and as a "pioneer in alternative medicine." He performs some 250 operations a year. The article notes that his "... Turkish roots influenced his sympathy for alternative medicine" because in Turkey families play a much larger role in the recuperation of sick relatives.

INVISIBLE DIVISIONS AND ZONES

Our body . . . this world . . . and the whole universe . . . are made up of different invisible zones and regions. These are guidelines which help us to find a certain location, as well as assist us with placement and arrangement.

There are five great divisions of the earth which are imaginary lines parallel to the equator and zoned according to biogeography such as temperature, light, prevailing plants, and animal life. There are time zones, which we consult before placing a long distance call to another part of the world; there are sports zones, dividing particular areas on a playing field; there are towns and cities which divide certain areas of land into commercial or residential zones; there are the oceans and sky which have zones for navigating boats and planes so they can find their way in the dark and through the fog.

Let's look at body divisions and zones. These guidelines are significantly important to the reflexologist because they help explain the connection between the reflex areas and the body parts to which they correspond.

- The Divisions . . . The human body has five main divisions which are parallel to the waistline (liken to the earth's five divisions which are parallel to the equator). The foot also has five transverse body divisions that help us distinguish which region of the body a particular part of the foot corresponds to.
- The Zones . . . When a sore spot on the foot is reflexed, it sends an invisible current of energy, which travels like a sound wave, up through the zones; if the pathways are clear, the foot feels no pain. But if the pathway is blocked to a specific part of the body,

this invisible electro-wave of activity converts the reflex stimulation into signals that feel like someone is pricking the foot with a pin.

Disturbance (of congestion or stress) at any point along a zone will have damaging effects on the natural energy flow within that zone. When pressure is applied to a "sore reflex," circulation is awakened within the zone and blood and lymph within the systems start to reactivate.

The important transportation network becomes energized and starts taking waste products away from the cells, carrying them to disposal sites of the body such as the lungs, liver, and kidneys. Then, as renewed circulation is accelerated, blood is able to nourish all the cells of the body with needed nutrients to help rebuild tissue, antibodies to fight disease, oxygen to produce energy, and hormones to regulate the internal chemistry of the body. This in turn will rebalance the body's various systems, so they can all work in harmony and function properly to help the body heal itself and alleviate all discomfort or illness.

Reflexology is like a sound wave that travels across the room: it is invisible, yet the auditory effect fills up the whole room. (Reflex energy is invisible, yet it balances the whole body.)

The body, like the world, also has many divisions and zones. Study charts F and G to increase your understanding of how proper stimulation of reflex areas on the feet reinforces energy stimulation along these invisible divisions and zones within the body.

CHAPTER 4

The Basics
of Successful
Reflexology

One excellent way to work the reflexes naturally is to follow the course of those who dwelt upon the earth many centuries ago. Remove your shoes and stockings and go about barefooted every chance you get.

We have influenced many of our friends, neighbors, students, and associates to adopt this habit of removing footwear when gardening, strolling around their yards, or simply while working or playing in the house.

THE IDEAL ENVIRONMENT

The ideal environment, of course, is in the great outdoors. Get out in the country as often as possible. Walk on the bare earth. Walk on rocks and sticks as nature intended that man should do. Be sure that the feet are *bare* so the electrical vibrations of the earth can be absorbed into the body, stimulating every living cell to renewed life and vitality.

Whenever one camps, goes up to the mountains, or down to the seashore, it would be most advantageous to go without footwear as much as possible. Walking on big rocks or small pebbles, in the sand or on the damp grass, all stimulate the reflexes in your feet.

It is wise to hunt for rocks deliberately, and walk on them. Hurt? Of course it will, especially if the walker has some sluggish, diseased parts of the body, or sick cells that are in need of a fresh supply of blood.

The rocks will press on sore reflexes, stimulating them, breaking up crystal deposits, and allowing blood to flow freely again, washing away sluggishness and poisons.

Did you ever notice how quickly water freshens when good water is poured into muddy water? Never forget that good circulation is the essence of a healthful life. Stagnation leads to untimely death. Just as a pond would soon become filled with algae and moss, eventually forming a hard crust, so will one's bloodstream, if a free, satisfactory circulation of blood is denied the cells and glands of all parts of the body.

Children should be encouraged to remove shoes and socks. Plans should be made for trips to the seashore, mountains, or out in the country. The entire family needs to walk over rough terrain, never avoiding sticks and stones. (Always with caution and proper supervision of children.) This can be turned into a game, the winner being the one who has come upon the most of these natural reflexers!

But let us presume that there will be families who, for one reason or another, are not able to get out in the country. How can they give themselves a natural reflex without the aid of nature?

There is a very effective tool now on the market which is called the "Deluxe-Foot-Roller." It can be used conveniently in the privacy of one's own home or while the user is otherwise occupied, for it can be placed on the floor while one is standing or sitting. (See Photo 3.) It is extremely helpful for those who cannot reach their own feet comfortably.

The principle of the foot roller is the same as that of the sticks and stones, only it can be used on the precise reflex points needed for a rewarding stimulation.

Accompanying the Deluxe-Foot-Roller is a chart explaining in detail where each reflex is in the feet and hands, which corresponds with important glands and organs in the body. It is possible to decide which parts of the body need stimulating by simply working the reflexes in the feet.

It is well to be aware that the kidneys will invariably need attention, for the poison released from dealing with any other part of the

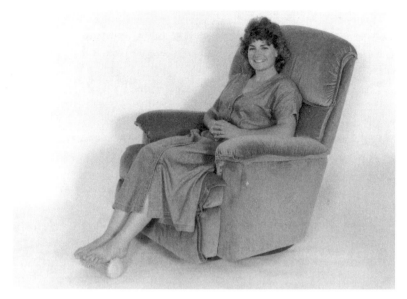

Photo 3. A comfortable position for using the Deluxe-Foot-Roller, to encourage renewed circulation to all energy zones.

body through reflexology will put extra labor on the kidneys. They comprise the filter system of the body and are to be stimulated last so they will be in condition for this extra burden put upon them.

The first few times the Deluxe-Foot-Roller is used, the treatment should be done cautiously. Too much poison flowing into the system at once can result in making one feel temporarily ill.

LEARNING THE BASICS

Length of Reflexology Session

A reflex session should always start with a few minutes of relaxing techniques, followed by the actual reflex workout.

The beginning reflex workout for a *specific disorder* should not extend over five minutes on each foot the first day. (This does not include time spent on relaxing techniques.)

If there is *no specific disorder*, the beginning workout should start with ten minutes of reflex work on each foot.

The discomfort resulting from a longer session would do no harm, but it could prove discouraging to any continuation of the reflex work. The general good will be inevitable, relaxing the nerves, stimulating veins, balancing the endocrine glands, and aiding the diaphragm.

You should first study the charts thoroughly, learning where the reflexes are in the feet, thus enabling you to diagnose your own illnesses. By becoming efficient in working the feet, locating tender spots, and referring to the charts, you will know what gland in your body is in special need of stimulation.

Reflexology is the natural way back to health.

Location of the Reflexes

It is important to study the reflex charts (see Chapter 2) since they will enable you to comprehend the relationship of reflex points to correlating parts of the body. These reflexes are not *in* the skin, but *under* it. Some are in an area as large as a lima bean. Others are no bigger than the head of a pin, so at times, one must press sufficiently hard to find them. Sometimes considerable searching is involved at first.

As you familiarize yourself with the location of reflexes, you will be able to mentally visualize the parts of the body to which they correspond.

How to Locate Reflexes

The reflexes can aptly be termed "buttons," for working them is not unlike pressing a button. Let us presume you did not feel well, but you did not know exactly where you felt ill. You would get out your hand probe, or even use your fingers or a rubber pencil eraser. You would press gently, but firmly, on the bottom of one foot, using a rotating motion, hunting for the button that would send back a message of tenderness or actual pain. This would indicate a congested area not receiving a full flow of life-giving blood in the corresponding part of the body.

You would then refer to your charts to discover what part of the body is sending you this summons for help. Next you would work the button for a few seconds. Don't be alarmed by the pain, and never press with such force that the tiny capillaries might be injured.

It will be a revelation when you realize how nature aids you in knowing where and how hard to use these reflex techniques for best results. Always approach the treatment gradually.

The entire foot should be reflexed in order not to miss any of the buttons waiting to give out distress signals. Each time one such button is located, it is to receive a brief, gentle, and thorough work-out.

Go to the other foot and repeat the procedure. Never be guilty of taking only half a treatment. You would not be satisfied with the work of an electrician who came and repaired one socket in your home which had become corroded but neglected other, perhaps more important areas. Another example is the battery of your car. If the cable is corroded, there will be no spark. When the corrosion is broken loose and sanded off, the cable can make a direct contact and the car comes to life. There is spark where needed, *unless* other places in the cable are similarly afflicted.

So it is, when you find a *corroded button* in the bottom of your foot. Start working it, press around and around, or back and forth, aware that you are wearing away the corrosion which has slowed the circulation to a certain portion of your body, making it impossible to work as perfectly as it was made to do.

When using the Deluxe-Foot-Roller on the floor, it will be easy to press the buttons that are tender and to find the buttons which are giving you trouble. (See Photo 3.)

The hand Reflex Roller is also excellent for this. (See Photo 4.)

Reflex Remote Control

Pressure on a certain button in the foot can result in an odd tingling sensation in quite another part of the body, and you will know that the reflex button has connected with this remote part. You then have proof that the healing message of the reflex is getting through to the source of trouble.

Sometimes the tingling will be in a part of the body where you least expect it, and this is encouraging. You have discovered a life-giving current of health! It is this reward which makes reflexology of such value. It covers all parts of the body and brings them under control.

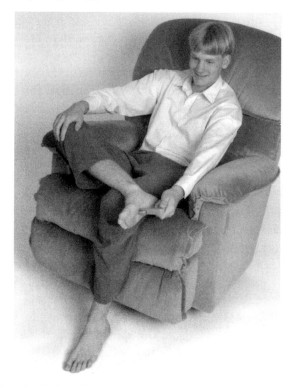

Photo 4. The simplicity of using the Reflex Roller makes reflexology fun and helps promote good health naturally.

It keeps any corrosion from forming and causing trouble at a later time.

The Roller Reflex is good for working on the upper parts of the feet, and the legs.

Having located a tender spot, be sure that the tenderness remains apparent as you continue the treatment. If it is tender only in the first instant of contact, you may be sure you have either gotten off the spot or are not pressing as hard on it as you should be.

BASIC POINTS TO PONDER

Be persistent and work all the reflexes with interest and sincere dedication. If one technique seems uncomfortable, or tiring to you or your reflex partner, try another. Keep in mind that each person is unique in size, disposition, and character, and each has a different threshold of pain or discomfort.

So remember that your aim is to stimulate renewed circulation, to send a charge of vital life force surging through the body, to open clogged pathways, to increase circulation and promote renewed health and vitality for yourself and each individual you wish to help with reflexology.

How Long to Work the Reflexes

Avoid working on one reflex very long, especially at first. Go from one sore spot to another, alternating often. When you return to a spot treated earlier, you will usually find that much of the tenderness has already left, at times even vanished completely. In other cases it may take several sessions for the painful reflex to be completely worked out.

You will know from your charts that the reflexes to the kidneys are found in the center of each foot. Since so much depends on them in this cleansing process, beware of overworking the reflex of this area. For best results give those important organs a chance to carry off the poisons without rushing this form of reflexology too quickly.

If congestion is bad and of long standing, each foot should probably not be worked any longer than five minutes the first time reflexology is used. Skip a day, then reflex perhaps ten minutes on each foot until you are able to detect less tenderness. As improvements in health are noted, use reflexology twice a week, fifteen minutes each foot; continue the schedule until the pain is completely gone.

The patient must keep in mind that he or she has been a long time getting in this current condition. Nature must be given a chance to correct this, although often the improvement is so rapid it does seem like a miracle.

What to Do When You Find a Very Sore Spot

If the reflex is very sore, a feather touch is enough to start; move on to other reflexes and every so often return to the *very sore spot*, and work it a few seconds (not so gently each time) until all soreness is gone. This may take several reflex sessions; do not overwork a very sore reflex.

Reflex Stages

The first stage of reflexology session is to relax the body and increase circulation. (It is best to begin your reflex work at a time when you can go to bed right afterward, or at least enjoy a nap, for reflexology is very relaxing.)

The second stage is to work out the sore spots.

The third stage is to give nature a chance to achieve balance and improve health *naturally*.

Use the Foot Reflexology Chart to Help Locate Reflex Areas

When you are learning, you may want to place the Foot Reflexology Chart next to the foot you are reflexing. This way, you can refer to it whenever you need help locating a reflex. You need to visualize the various body parts as you work on the foot. Remember you are not just *rubbing* the foot, but you are working reflexes under the skin, reflexes that will trigger impulses to normalize the whole body.

A Note of Caution

If there is an affliction that you are not sure about, check with a professional care provider before using reflexology. There may be certain maladies where it is best not used. Such an instance may occur when there are specific problems with a pregnancy because certain reflex points have a relaxing effect on the reproductive organs.

Also some doctors feel reflexology may complicate matters for cancer patients who are undergoing chemotherapy treatments.

Personally I have never had a negative experience with reflexology; however, it is not a substitute for medical care. Therefore, if you are suffering from a medical problem, seek qualified professional help.

LIFE'S VITAL ENERGY FORCE

All creation, heaven and earth come from a source of energy. Energy from the earth's vibrations causes earthquakes to tremble the crust of the earth, volcanoes to erupt, the mountains to push up, and the oceans to change their tides. There are energetic cells in the atmosphere which stimulate a natural movement of air forcing the winds and causing a change in the weather. These vital energy forces that flow through space and earth transform the planet we live on.

"Life energy" is the fuel of all living things. We all have energy circulating within our bodies. We are alive and constantly growing new cells. This circuit of *life's vital energy force*, started at the moment of conception, will circulate within our bodies as long as we live.

Vital Energy Cells

Our body is composed of trillions of living cells which have various shapes and sizes, and perform many different functions. Just as it takes all kinds of building materials to make a complete house—foundation, frame and its many parts, a water system and electrical outlets—so does it take all kinds of cells to completely make up (or build) the body's frame and its many parts, including blood cells and nerve cells to regulate its functions and actions.

The body's cells contain a chemical compound called ATP (adenosine triphosphate) which controls a very large part of your body. It helps the body to move, to process its functions, even helps it to think. Just as electricity keeps appliances working, ATP helps the body operate and is the "life energy" that keeps it alive.

Reflexology activates this very important life-giving current of energy to the cells, which helps keep them healthy. A reflex workout will stimulate life's vital energies, helping to improve circulation, reduce stress and tensions, and balance the condition of the cells so they can divide and reproduce to replace the old worn-out or injured cells. Study reflexology and the human body connection, because the best investment you can make in your life is learning how to stay healthy.

The Importance of Keeping the Cellular Level Balanced

Modern science tells us that the human body is made up of many accumulations of electro fields. When these fields become blocked, an imbalance within the system may occur, resulting in symptoms of mental or physical distress.

Many scientific studies have proven that imbalance within the body causes much sickness and disease. For instance, when energy is not circulating well, the internal systems become sluggish, and the entire circulatory system suffers. When the energy force flowing to the heart is not in proper balance, it may cause high or low blood pressure. An imbalance of the pancreas, rendering it unable to control the level of sugar in the blood, may result in high blood sugar "diabetes," or low blood sugar "hypoglycemia."

RECHARGE VITAL ENERGIES

The body is like a battery: It gets low on energy every now and then, and needs to be recharged. In a way stimulation to the reflexes is like this process. Working the reflexes relieves tensions and promotes renewed circulation to unblock vital energies. When the body regains its internal strength is has the power to heal itself, thus bringing effective relief from many ailments.

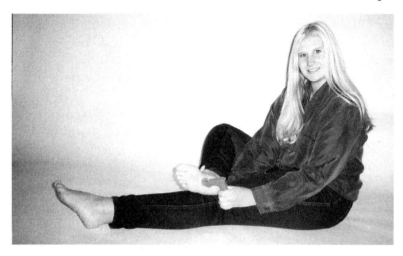

Photo 5. Foot reflexology is an easy and very effective technique to wake-up circulation and increase physical and mental energy.

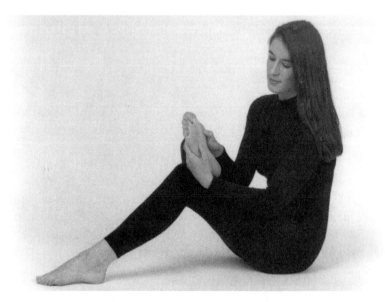

Photo 6. Benefit from the rewards of reflexology by finding a body stance that is right for you. For example, keep feet in same position as above and lie down on your back, place pillows under shoulders and head for added comfort and relaxation.

How to Use Basic Reflexology Techniques

Various reflex techniques are easy to learn and will provide the essentials you need for doing reflexology. After you learn the basic steps, they will most likely become very natural for you to use. You can practice the various methods on yourself before you do reflexology on another person. This will help you focus on the pressure you are using and get a better understanding of the invigorating effects.

Always remember that reflexology is nature's way to perfect health. It is free for you to learn and use, to safeguard your health and prevent illness. Once you have mastered the basics you can be creative and develop your own personal style.

Keep in mind that reflexology is a method of alternating pressure to various reflex areas to help the body maintain balance. Each reflex area on the foot corresponds to a specific gland, organ, nerve, or structure in the body. Your goal is to help nature soothe away stress and tension, release blockages that inhibit life's energy flow, and restore normal circulation.

In this chapter you will learn how to use your fingers and thumbs to "work" the reflexes. You will also learn various "holding" methods that you can use when applying your reflex skills to the feet. And we will highlight a few relaxing techniques that you can use before and after a reflex workout. These techniques are very effective in helping people to relax. Reflexology will be easier to learn if you first study the charts and techniques; however, do not try to absorb all the information at once. Just learn a little now and a little more later, taking it gradually, one step at a time.

EVERYBODY CAN BENEFIT FROM LEARNING REFLEXOLOGY

Learning reflexology also helps you understand more about your body and how it functions. You will find that you feel more centered, and you will soon start thinking of other ways to keep your body healthy, such as combining movement and exercise with proper breathing, and watching your diet. As you discover how beneficial reflexology is in attaining a healthy new self-awareness, you will also learn to appreciate the wonder of yourself!

With this knowledge about helping yourself will also come the realization that you can help others. Your wish to help a friend or a family member will soon be a reality. This is when reflexology really becomes exciting!

Every person can benefit from learning reflexology skills. These techniques can be used today or any time in the future to help relieve specific ailments and to increase mental and physical energy.

By learning the proper reflex techniques, applying them correctly and giving nature a chance to promote deep relaxation and healing, you will be helping yourself and others to regain good health *naturally*.

HOW TO USE YOUR THUMBS AND FINGERS CORRECTLY

Reflexology will be easier for you to do if you learn the proper way to use your thumbs and fingers. Here are several simple illustrations with written explanations of how to "work" the reflexes. You want to have confidence in your skills, so concentrate on learning these techniques, then practice using them until they become easy for you.

Finding the "Working" Part of Your Thumb

Using your thumb properly will contribute to the overall efficiency of your reflex work. It is important that you use your thumb in a certain way, so that you can effectively reach into the reflex points.

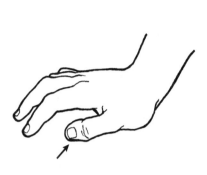

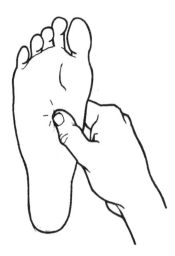

Illustration 1a. To find the "working" part of your thumb, place your hand down lightly on this book. Notice the medial (inside) edge of the thumb and how it touches the surface of the book?

Illustration 1b. With thumb bent at first joint, use the "working" edge to apply pressure on a reflex, and it will give a needle-point contact with the tender area. Always make sure that your thumbnail is well trimmed to prevent the nail from pressing into the foot.

Learning the Proper Technique to "Thumb-Walk"

Now you will learn to use your thumb for "walking" along a reflex area that extends over one-half inch on the foot. This technique is used often; you can use it when working the reflex to a large organ, such as the liver or lungs, and it works well when criss-crossing over a whole region. You can also use this movement when working up or down a zone, such as for the spine.

For this, you will bend the first joint of the thumb, using a very small range of motion, bend your thumb at the first joint and travel forward, like an inchworm. This may be practiced on the palm and forearm of your hand with the opposite thumb, to good advantage. And in this way you can get the feel of the amount of pressure to use. It may take a little time at first; however, you will be able to develop the proper technique with some practice.

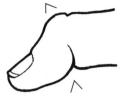

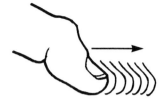

Illustration 2a. Slightly bend your thumb at the first joint. You do not want it to be straight, or it will not move appropriately.

Illustration 2b. Walk your thumb forward like a tiny inchworm, first by bending at the first joint . . . then press down on the reflex point . . . move thumb forward slightly . . . and repeat. Keep your thumb bent and in contact with flesh; move it approximately seven times within one inch of space on the foot.

Learning the Proper Technique to "Finger-Walk"

When doing the "Finger-Walk" you will use one or more fingers; usually the index and middle fingers work best. Make your fingers flex-

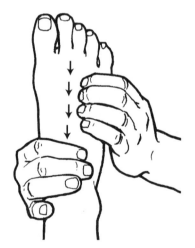

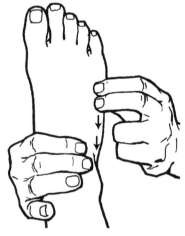

Illustration 3a. Finger-walk on top of foot by placing fingers on top and thumb on the sole side for support. With fingers together, apply pressure and pull back, "walking" them from the toes toward the leg. Make several trips to cover all reflexes on top of the foot.

Illustration 3b. Finger-walk along the side of foot by taking very small steps forward, press in, and slightly pull back. Change hands and finger-walk down the other side of foot.

able for working by slightly bending them at the first and middle joints. Use very small "inchworm-size steps" as you walk your fingers on the foot. Support foot with opposite hand, placing thumb on the other side of foot for leverage. Keep the pressure steady and work with slow smooth motions. This technique is great for working on the top or sides of the feet.

How to Use the "Press-and-Roll" Technique

When explaining how to work a reflex area, we often tell our students to use either "a pressing, rolling motion," or "a rolling, circular motion." This is a very popular technique that almost everyone likes to use. Position your thumb and fingers correctly (see page 45 and 46)

Take your foot (or a companion's foot) in one hand and press with the edge of your thumb. Press-and-roll in a circular motion, as if you were trying to crumble a hard bread crumb with your thumb. Keeping your thumb in contact with the foot, apply steady pressure. A very simple and easy-to-use method which works well on almost all reflex areas, you can even use it when pinpointing a very small reflex point, such as the pituitary or pineal reflex.

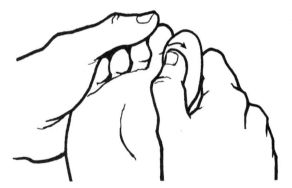

Illustration 4. Press-and-roll the "working" part of the thumb into the reflex; apply steady pressure as you slowly rotate your thumb on the pressure point.

Developing the "Press and Pull-Down" Technique

You can use this technique where the skin is hard, such as the heel, or on a specific small point such as the appendix reflex. Bend your

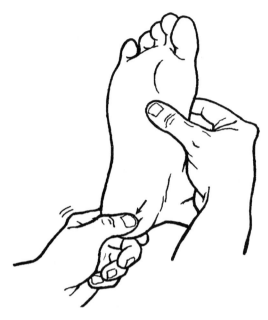

Illustration 5. Press and pull-down along the edge of heel. Work around the heel to improve circulation.

thumb at the first joint and place the working edge on the reflex. Press the thumb into the reflex point, and pull down sharply. Hold for a moment, let up on the pressure, then press in again and pull the thumb down. Repeat three times, then release.

EFFECTIVE REFLEX TECHNIQUES

Reflexology techniques are easy to learn; and once you know the actual pressure points, then you will find that the routine will be pretty much the same for each person. Of course chronically ill people should not receive long sessions to start, and you will want to be very gentle because their reflexes will be extremely tender. In contrast, those who are strong and healthy will probably take longer sessions, and you will need to apply more pressure.

Small children or pregnant women may require special care. Be sensitive to and considerate of their personal needs. A tender touch is recommended.

How Much Pressure to Use

The manner in which you work depends on sensitivity and depth of the reflex. Use a gentle touch, yet exert enough pressure to stimulate renewed circulation. Use from one to ten pounds of pressure on the thumb against the foot. Your intuition will help you decide the right amount; the more experience you get, the easier it will be for you.

How to Properly Support the Foot

Whether doing reflexology on yourself or another person, you should use two hands for additional strength. Proper holding techniques give you more endurance and provide a method of moving the foot so that the reflex areas are easier to reach. You can give support to the foot by placing the fingers of one hand behind or around the foot you are working on. You can also hold one hand beneath the foot or wrap fingers around the toes to help keep the foot steady. This will support the foot, and give your thumb or fingers on the opposite hand increased pressure power.

A Few Relaxing Techniques

When you first start a reflex session it is helpful to use at least one relaxing technique before you proceed with the workout in order to loosen up tension. Relaxing methods are also beneficial at the end of each session. Here are a few easy methods that you can use, or you can create your own techniques. Use great caution when rotating the ankles and toes, especially when working on stiff, arthritic, swollen, or disfigured feet. Always relax both feet. You will find other helpful relaxing routines throughout the book.

Foot Rotation   Place one hand under heel for support, and the other hand around either side of the foot. (Right hand will hold right side of foot, left hand will hold left side.) Gently rotate at ankle clockwise a few times, then counter-clockwise a few times. The foot may be stiff or tight; never force it to move, just gently try to sway it at first. Also be careful not to dig your fingers in under the ankle area. Rotating the foot is wonderful for stimulating the lymphatic system for renewed circulation. It is good for both increasing energy and relaxing the body, whichever the person needs.

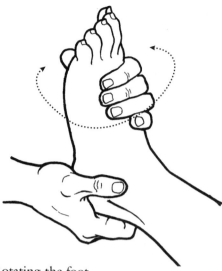

Illustration 6a. Rotating the foot.

Toe Rotations   Support foot with one hand. With the other hand, place thumb on the bottom of toe, use index and middle fingers on top at mid-joint; slightly move with a gentle upward movement. Using mild traction, rotate each toe separately, and in both directions.

After you have rotated toes; place hand over them, thumb on bottom side and fingers over the top of foot. Rotate all toes at once; extend upward and to the left a few times, then repeat to the right. These techniques are used to relax tension and loosen up muscles.

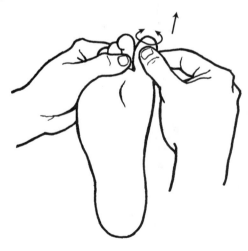

Illustration 6b. Rotating the toes.

Press-and-Slide Place both thumbs on the sole of foot, fingers on top. Use a press-and-slide action with thumb and fingers moving upward and going off the sides of foot with a gentle pinching movement. Starting near the heel, use alternating hands and continue upwards to the toes. Repeat several times. Work both top and bottom of each foot; and press hard enough so that you do not tickle the foot. This technique is good for increasing circulation and promoting relaxation.

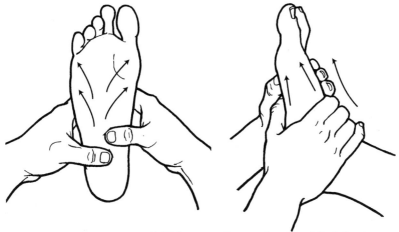

Illustration 7a. Press-and-Slide upwards.

Illustration 7b. Work both top and bottom of each feet.

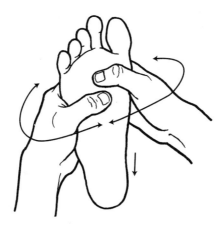

Illustration 7c: "Hugging" the Feet Wrap your hands around the sides of one foot. Thumbs on sole, fingers laced over top. Gently press the foot with your hands, starting with a gentle squeeze around the

toes and work down to the heel. "Hug" both the tops, bottoms, and sides of each foot. This not only feels wonderful, but it is great for loosening tight muscles and helps relax the nerves.

TAKE CARE OF YOURSELF

There are various positions that you can use when learning self-help reflexology. We will highlight a few on the following pages, before you start mastering the reflex work, acquired from Part Two. (The suggested positions for working on your family and friends will be covered in Part Three.)

First you must pay close attention to your body and, when reflexing your feet, *listen to what the tender spots are telling you.* A painful reflex may suggest a threatening health problem. This is the time to stimulate or "work" the tender reflexes and allow healing energy to alleviate the effects of stress or congestion. As the tension is cleared, renewed energy and circulation will flow freely throughout the system; toxins and impurities can now be flushed out, circulation improves, and the whole body returns to a state of optimal health and remarkable balance.

Continue to have patience with your body's healing process. Remember it may have taken a long time to get into this condition, so allow it time to heal.

Go slowly in the beginning, and be careful not to overwork the reflexes. Your goal is to relax tension and tone up the body first; then harmony and renewed health will be restored naturally.

Comfort Is Important

When reflexing *your own* feet, you will want to use a variety of positions. Find those that are comfortable for you and give you good access to reflexes. You may like the foundation of the floor, or you can use your favorite easy chair, place a few pillows around you for support. You may like to do self-help reflex techniques on your feet while in the comfort of your own bed. You decide which position is best for you to use. Always use the one that is most comfortable to you. Remember you must be relaxed to dissolve stress and tension.

Working Your Own Reflexes

Whether you are learning reflexology for individual use or to help another person, you should work your own reflexes first to get a general idea of the amount of pressure to apply. Working on your own feet is also a good method of practicing your techniques. Find a comfortable location where you can reach your feet without strain. Stimulate the tops, sides, and bottoms of both feet to send healing energy through the body and help restore youthful vitality. (see Photo 7.)

Another method is to support the foot being worked by resting it on the opposite thigh or knee. Use one or both hands to work the reflexes. (see Photo 8.)

When doing self-help reflexology, it is very important to get yourself into a comfortable position. For some, working the reflexes from bed is comfortable. Use pillows for added support. You can lie on your back with one foot resting on opposite bent knee. Or lie on side with knees bent, so that you can reach your feet.

Pillows are also a good method of leverage, and work well when you are in a sitting positin or lying down. (see Photo 9.) Look for various self-help positions in Part Two.

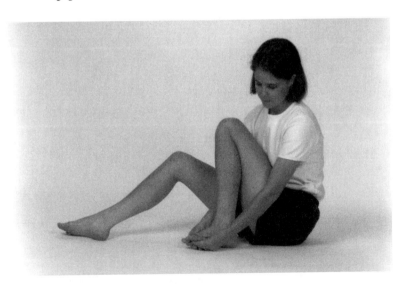

Photo 7. Stimulate reflexes with foot in front of you.

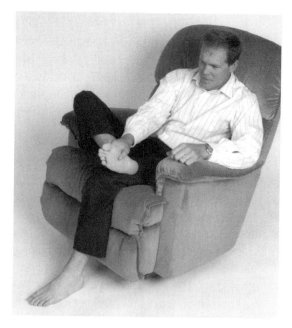

Photo 8. Sit comfortably with foot resting on knee.

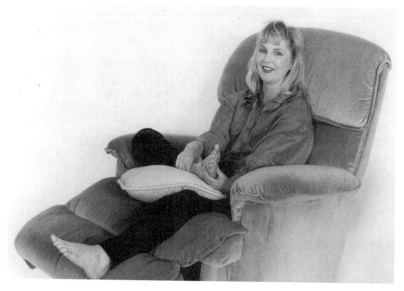

Photo 9. Rest in a cozy chair, or on the sofa, and use pillows to help support your leg and foot.

Self-Help Tools

During one of Dr. Fitzgerald's lectures, *A Key to Zone Therapy*, he stated, "Professional operators and doctors find the thumb 'wears out' too quickly and becomes tender." He went on to say that many operators were using modern tools instead of the hand, as these tools often do deeper and finer work than the thumb will do.

Of course it is great when there is someone there to give you reflexology. But consider the times when no one is available to help you. Well, this is the time you need to take care of yourself. You must not wait until illness strikes. Self-help reflexology will provide you with an instant, natural approach to keeping yourself healthy, by helping your body to balance with inner healing forces so that it will function at its fullest potential.

With the aid of specially designed, simple-to-use reflex tools, almost anyone can be helped by reflexology. Safe and inexpensive tools make reflexing easy for people with arthritis, weak or tired fingers or those who otherwise could not experience the benefits of renewed circulation. These tools help give fingers additional strength, to work out the tender spots, and are effective for energizing the circulation to benefit cellular development in all areas of the body. Another aid, the Deluxe-Foot-Roller, is very effective for those who cannot reach their own feet.

(An order form is provided at the back of this book.)

HELPING YOURSELF WITH REFLEXOLOGY

GUIDE-AT-A-GLANCE

Visual guides are located throughout Part Two to help you recognize where various glands and organs are in the body, and where their corresponding reflex is located in the feet.

For example, the first illustration shows that the reflex points in the toes relate to those in the head.

CHAPTER 6

Reflexology of the Toes

Location of
HEAD and NECK
in the body.

Corresponding
HEAD and NECK
reflexes.

There is no portion of your wonderfully constructed foot which does not have its part to play in reflexology. The foot offers a new, unique way to health through its reflex therapy. I shall detail how to apply the simple and natural method of working the reflex points on your own feet for a new way to attain vibrant health.

You have now studied the charts and have a general idea of how each different part of your body has a corresponding reflex located some place on the feet, and how and where to locate them.

You have found a position in which you are comfortable and relaxed while reaching each foot easily.

You understand the gentle, deep, circular pressing motion that you must use to reach these reflexes correctly. If you don't reach the inner reflex button it will not be able to send a stimulation to the distressed part of the body, nor will you be able to break up the accumulated crystals in the capillaries.

PINPOINTING THE PITUITARY REFLEX

You are ready for your first experience in the vitalizing, rejuvenating method of reflexology. You will now learn how to use reflexology on your own feet.

Take your left foot in your left hand and with the fingers of the right hand press the big toe gently all over. Do you feel any tender spots? If not, then press a little harder with a circular motion. This is just so you can get the feel of it.

We will start by working the hypothalamus and pituitary reflexes in the center of the big toe, since these are the most important glands that we have. They are located so close to each other in the brain, that when you reflex one, you will also reflex the other. Together they control body growth, blood pressure, heartbeat, and regulate the activities of all other glands. (See Photo 10.)

Sending new stimulation to this gland in the young or old will grant a new lease on life. Notice in Photo 11 how the instrument is pressed into the center pad on the big toe. I don't believe that you can find this reflex with the fingers unless it is extremely tender. Although the spot is no larger than the head of a pin, touching it in the act of reflexing is like sticking a pin in the toe. This is especially true with older people whose circulation to the pituitary has been cut down for many years. Age is not always a factor, however, since many young people have deficient pituitaries.

Especially in men, the reflexes may be very deep and the pressure will have to be equally deep. Here the small Magic Reflexer or the Reflex Hand Probe is especially helpful. If not available, try a pencil with a new eraser. Now press the probe into the soft pad of the big toe in the very center. (Look for the widest part on either side of your toe;

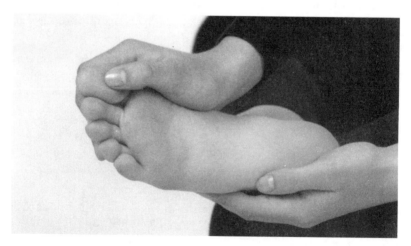

Photo 10. Working the reflex to the hypothalamus and pituitary glands.

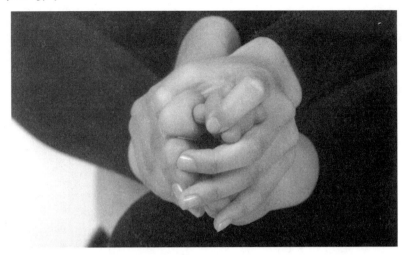

Photo 11. Using the Magic Reflexer to pinpoint deep reflex points in the big toe.

you can pinpoint this reflex point at the center of this wide area.) Keep pressing with a little, rotating motion. If you don't feel a sharp stab of pain, either you are not on the reflex point or you are not pressing deeply enough. Be careful not to bruise the tender capillaries in the skin while doing this. When you feel a sharp pain, then you are on the reflex to the pituitary gland. Having found it, work it with a gentle, circular motion for two or three seconds the first time.

You will find that there will usually be more tenderness in the reflex of the pituitary on one foot than on the other. In this case you will find that most of the reflexes on this particular foot will be more tender than on the other foot, especially the reflexes to the endocrine glands. This will indicate that there is more congestion or malfunctioning of one or more glands or organs on this side of the body, giving you a clue to follow, and enabling you to help relieve many ailments in a shorter period of time.

The Link Between the Hypothalamus and the Pituitary

The pituitary is controlled by a part of the brain, the hypothalamus. The hypothalamus directs hormone production, while the pituitary gland produces the "Master Hormones" which regulate the other glands.

The hypothalamus is attached to the pituitary and controls its secretions. Together both glands manufacture 16 or more various hormones. The pituitary, crucial to both the nervous and the endocrine systems, releases many hormones that affect our development.

When you reflex the center of each big toe, you send an electro-wave of activity to both the hypothalamus and the pituitary, to revitalize the energy needed for your hormones to carry their messages directly to your cells.

Pineal Gland

You are also near the reflex to the pineal gland (the pituitary helper) which, as you can see in Charts A and B, is located near the center of the brain. So the reflexes to the pineal would be located near the center of the big toe, just a tiny bit toward the second toe and a bit up toward the tip of the toe. Try finding this spot by the same method you used in locating the reflex to the pituitary gland. Work it for a few seconds with a gentle, circular motion.

This pineal gland is located behind the hypothalamus and pituitary gland in the brain. After you work the center of the big toe, work slightly above, below, and around the toe to stimulate other reflexes to the brain.

Now put your left foot on the floor and pick up the right foot in the same position you just used on the left, taking the right foot in the right hand and reflexing the big toe with the fingers of the left hand. Next, take the reflex probe and press it into the center of the pad of the big toe, working it around until you feel the sharp pain that tells you that you are pressing on the pituitary reflex. Work it for a few seconds no matter how painful it is. Sometimes you only need to touch it two or three seconds the first time to get results. Then find the pressure point to the pineal and work as you did on the left foot. This also may be quite painful, but this is all the more reason it needs stimulation. You will be amazed how quickly the soreness will work out of the reflexes to these three glands—sometimes in only two or three sessions.

Put your right foot back on the floor and lift the left foot back into position. Changing legs often keeps them from becoming too cramped by holding them in one position for a long time. After awhile the muscles will become accustomed to these positions and you will not need to change legs as often.

ADDITIONAL TECHNIQUES FOR THE TOES

Let's continue to work on the big toe. Remember, the left foot represents the left side of the body, so when we perform work on the big toe of the left foot we are contacting the reflexes to the left side of the head. Take the big toe in the fingers of the right hand and reflex it with a pressing, rotating motion covering the whole toe. You will probably find several tender spots at first; reflex them gently for a few seconds.

WORKING THE REFLEXES TO THE NOSE, TEETH/GUMS/JAWS

Notice in Photo 12 how the thumb is pressing just below the toenail on the top of the foot. Reflexes found on the top of the toes generally go to areas on the front side of the face, such as the nose. Therefore, by sending energy through zone 1, on top of the toe, you can help speed healing to relieve a sore nose. (See Chart D on pg. 11) You would work both big toes toward the instep. Of course you know

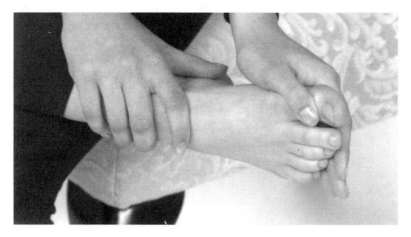

Photo 12. Stimulating the reflexes on top of the big toe.

that both big toes (and both thumbs) are in zone 1 which goes vertically through the center of the head and body. As we work the four smaller toes, we are "fine-tuning" the multitude of head reflexes also reflected on the soles. Each reflex stays within the same zone as the corresponding part of the head.

For teeth, gum, and jaw problems, you would work all five toes on both feet. Each person has an individualized bone structure and would, therefore, need to visually align his or her own teeth and jaws within the respective zone area. These reflexes will be found on the same side of the body as the discomfort.

For instance, if your left front tooth ached, you would work on the top of the left big toe, because they are both in the same zone, on the same side of the body. If the back right molar hurt, you would work the fourth or fifth toe (whichever zone your molar is in) on the right foot.

To work this area, use your index finger and thumb to slowly press-and-roll the toe within the painful zone. Holding pressure on the whole toe (toenail and sole side) for five to seven minutes, will produce an anesthetic effect in the corresponding painful area of the zone.

NECK REFLEXES

As we move on down the toe toward the foot, we find the reflexes on the bottom of the toe at the basal joint (where the toe joins the foot) to be the reflexes to the neck. Notice here how the bones of the big toe connect to those of the foot, and how they resemble the bones of the cervical (neck) vertebrae, which Chart C illustrates.

The outside basal joint of the big toe (next to the second toe) has the reflexes to the outer side of the neck, while the inside (medial side of toe) contains those to the center of the neck.

THROAT AND TONSIL REFLEXES

Even though we learned that the throat and face reflexes are represented on the top of the feet (anterior side of body), we also know that all reflex points are mirrored on the soles of the feet (see Chart B).

When working reflexes to the face, throat, thyroid, or tonsil, we get a much greater response from applying pressure to points on the bottom of the feet. Also work the basal joints of the big toe, where it fastens onto the foot. In case of a sore throat, you will find this very tender. Reflexing all the way around the big toe and fine tuning smaller toes is also beneficial.

Check the Lymphatic System

In any cases of problems with the nose, throat, or ears, always check the lymph reflexes for tenderness, as there could be an infection in these areas. Check the neck for swollen lymph nodes to see if there is a blockage. If one side of the neck is swollen, work the lymph reflexes in the foot on the same side of the body first; then repeat on the opposite foot to make sure circulation of the lymph fluid is doing its job of flushing out poisons and toxins.

Also work the reflex areas to the other organs that remove wastes from the body such as the liver and the kidneys.

Case of Sore Throat Healed

One day a neighbor came to me saying her three-year-old son was suffering with a sore throat. His fever was very high. Returning home with her, I rubbed the reflexes to the child's throat (the underside of the big toe). Because of the fever, I also worked the reflexes to the pituitary gland, in the center of the big toe. Later in the day, I saw him out playing in the snow!

Incidentally, children are the most willing subjects for reflexology and appear to crave it instinctively. Many whom I know are given to urging their mothers to call me instead of a doctor when they are ill.

In summation, if there is tenderness anywhere on the big toe, there is tension and congestion which must be released in the interest of good health.

HEADACHES AND EYE WEAKNESS

Tension in the neck causes many headaches and eye weaknesses. So, after working the entire big toe, relax the stress in this area of the neck by taking the big toe between the thumb and index finger and rotating it in a circular motion, first to the left, then to the right. Loosen all toes by pulling and turning them slightly. Never force a toe to move; turn it until it resists slightly, then rotate in opposite direction. Gently rotate and stretch each toe to promote improved circulation.

This may take a few reflex sessions, but the results will be especially gratifying. It is as if someone held your head in his or her hands and gently rotated it in a similar manner; only this method of limbering the cervical (neck) vertebrae through the big toe will give better results.

If your leg feels tired, change positions again and work on the toe of the right foot before we proceed.

Now that you have worked both big toes in zone 1, let's move on to the toe next to it, the second toe, in zone 2. Between these two toes, close to where they join the foot, more at the basal joint of the second toe, there is a reflex we call the "pain eliminator." This special button stops many headaches, colds and helps calm stress.

Often a tenderness here is noticed on only one foot, because nerves on that side of the neck may be pinched, or circulation is blocked. Reflexing here can be most rewarding in relieving headaches, in many cases when nothing else will help.

If you cannot find a tender spot here, and your headache is still throbbing, continue to stimulate the reflexes on all toes. Work the entire big toe, as well as all toes on both feet. Squeeze the balls of your toes between your thumb and index finger, searching for sore spots (see Illustration 6b). Reflex the tips of all toes, and in between each toe; then rotate and stretch each toe in both directions to limber up the cervical vertebrae.

Many headaches are caused by a stressed back or a tight shoulder. If there is discomfort in the shoulder or along the spine, work the reflex corresponding to the area. For the back reflex, work up and down the instep on both feet. Read additional techniques about how to reflex your spine in Chapter 7. Work the outside of the foot, as well as below and all around the little toe, to loosen the muscles surrounding the shoulder.

There are several different types of headaches. Some can be brought on by tension, others from straining of the eyes, others from constipation, or by the upset of some organ such as the stomach or liver. In each case the reflex to the corresponding organ will be very tender and should be worked on in conjunction with the toes. I have never failed to relieve a headache with reflexology, even in cases of agonizing migraines.

REFLEXES OF THE EYES

At the bottom of the second and third (zones 2 and 3) toes, you will find the reflexes to the eyes. (See Chart B and also Photo 13.)

To work these reflexes, you hold the foot in position and press with a rolling motion just under these two toes. This is usually easy to do with your thumb, but in some cases you may find it more reward- ing to use the Reflex Probe or a like tool. Press and roll this area, searching for tender spots, and when you find them, work each one for a few seconds.

Many different cases of near blindness have been helped by working the reflexes in the feet. Not only are the direct eye reflexes responsible for eye disorders, but often there are taut nerves in the back of the neck which cause a normal blood supply to the head and eyes to be cut off. Also, remember that when there is an abnormal condition of the eyes, the functioning of the kidneys often appears to be a contributing factor. Therefore, working the kidney and adrenal reflexes is also very important.

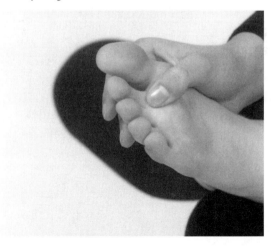

Photo 13. Work the reflexes under toes for relieving a headache, or trou- bles of the eyes, ears and sinuses.

EAR REFLEXES

Still holding the foot in the same position, let's go to the reflexes of the ears, which are in a position similar to the eye reflexes, only just under the next two toes, the fourth and fifth in zones 4 and 5. (See Chart B.) We will work these reflexes just as we did for the eyes, repeating the process in both directions several times. Keep in mind that the right foot governs the right ear, the left foot, the left ear. In the case of middle or inner ear troubles work zones 2 and 3, just below the eye reflexes. (See illustration on page 233.)

The taut nerves of the neck could have the same abnormal effect on the ears as they do on the eyes. Gently work the joints of all toes to loosen tightness, thus facilitating improved circulation.

Be aware that any tenderness needs appropriate work for it indicates that somewhere there is tension which needs release, or congestion which prevents the blood from flowing freely into the zone.

SINUS REFLEXES

Now let us go back to the position of the reflexes to the eyes and ears. You will find the reflexes to the sinuses by dropping down into the foot just a tiny bit below the eye and ear reflexes. Work them in the same manner that you worked the reflexes of the eyes and ears.

Reflex between all toes, but especially between the second and third toes where there seems to be a very definite reflex to the sinuses. After you find the tender spot in this area, you may work this reflex for several minutes, or until you can feel the congestion of the sinuses loosening up.

Rub the tips of each toe with the Reflex Probe or the thumbnail, by rolling either one across the top of each toe. This also tends to relieve sinus congestion. Now take each toe, one at a time, and give it two or three light twists and rolls for relaxing.

HOW TO REFLEX AFTER A STROKE OR HEAD INJURY

You just learned the guidelines to zone therapy, and how the body has invisible pathways that travel vertically up the body to the top of the head. You have learned the fundamental concept that when you are reflexing the feet to stimulate the body's flow of energy, the left foot

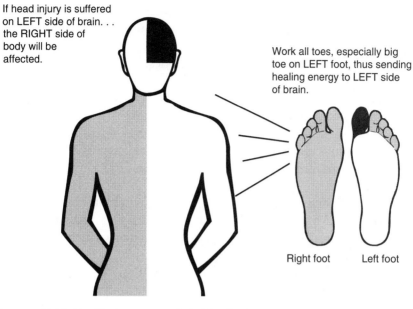

If head injury is suffered on LEFT side of brain. . . the RIGHT side of body will be affected.

Work all toes, especially big toe on LEFT foot, thus sending healing energy to LEFT side of brain.

Right foot   Left foot

Right side of body   Left side of body

Illustration 8. Effective Reflex technique to use after a stroke.

corresponds to the left side of the head, and the right foot to the right side of the head.

When the brain cells have been damaged due to a head injury, brain tumor or stroke, it will produce an effect on the ability to physically move certain parts on the *opposite* side of the body.

For example, if a stroke caused abnormality to the left side of the brain, parts of the body on the right side would be affected. This is because the left side of the brain interprets what the right side of the body will do, and vice versa.

(Therefore, if the right side of the body suffers paralysis, reflex the left big toe. This will stimulate the nerve fibers in the left brain, so that they can communicate to the right side of the body.)

Press the top and bottom side of the toe in various places searching for a tender spot. Also work the inner and outer sides of each big toe for best results in finding the sore reflex. Work tender spots with a pressing circular motion, as this may be the reflex to the part of the brain that caused the stroke.

Be sure that these areas are well worked until all tenderness is gone. A general coverage of the whole big toe, as well as "fine tuning" all other toes, is the surest method of effective reflex performance.

To encourage renewed circulation to the affected areas on the RIGHT side of the body, work the corresponding reflexes on RIGHT foot.

To minimize the risk of stroke episodes, work all reflex areas on both feet and to all toes to stimulate good circulation. Strokes are often caused by a blockage to the brain or oxygen deprivation to a particular area of the brain.

Recovery takes a lot of dedication and hard work, but damaged brain cells can learn new roles. Reflexology has helped many stroke victims to remarkable recoveries, especially those occurring in early childhood.

A letter came the other day from a lady who I am very proud of. She works hard to help herself which makes her a wonderful example for the rest of us. Let me share a part of her letter with you.

Reflexology and Prayer Restored Life

Dear Mrs. Carter,

I am a victim of aneurysm of the brain. Six years ago the surgeon closed my head after discovering that my brain was destroyed. I was left "brain dead," with very little hope of living and NO hope of regaining ANY part of my brain. He told my family that he did not expect me to live and, if I did, I would only be a living vegetable.

You speak of faith, and it was by faith that I was restored. Prayers went forth and I was restored to a healthy mind.

I have been having some bad pain in my leg and I showed my husband the reflex point and after a couple of times working it out, the pain was gone! I really thank God. Thank Him for teachers who help make life better.

I now have complete control of my right body use, while my left side has no movement. However, I have feeling in the left side of my body and I climb stairs, hang clothes (using my teeth to hold the sheets that are in my laundry.)

I have helped my children with their school lessons. Reflexology has already helped me to help my family, and I am looking forward to learning more about reflexology so that I might help others to regain health and tranquility.

—S.I.

Reflex Techniques for the Back and Spine

Location of SPINE in body.

Corresponding SPINAL reflex areas.

The spine's importance to general health is familiar to all practitioners. Osteopathic and chiropractic doctors understand that the greater part of one's well-being depends on the condition of the spine. To work the reflexes of the back or spine is to relax the muscle tension surrounding any vertebra that is not in perfect and healthful alignment.

You have studied the position of the spine and its reflexes in Chart B. Look at Illustration 9 for working the back and spine reflexes. Notice how the thumb of the right hand is pressing into the center of the instep of the right foot! This is where the reflex to the center of the spine is located, and the spot that the thumb is pressing would be a reflex to about the center of the back or the waistline.

Have your foot up in position. Now take the large toe, beginning in the middle of it. Remember the big toe represents the head and the neck. Now, feel the middle joint of the big toe for the first vertebra of the spine reflex. Follow these bones on down the foot with your thumb, and notice how the bones in the instep resemble the vertebrae in your back.

Relief of Back Tensions or Pain

If there is pain or tension in the upper part of the back, between the shoulders or around the neck, look for tenderness at basal joint and

71

just below the large toe. If there is backache in the center of the back, then look for tenderness in the middle of the foot, around the waistline area. If you have lower back trouble, then follow the inner side of the foot down to the heel. Use the pressing, rolling motion along these bones in the foot to search out the tender spots.

Press slightly in and under the bones of the foot, especially in the area just above the heel, which is the lower lumbar region, shown in Charts C and H.

The whole spinal column is located in the exact center of the body, so the reflexes will cover the entire area along the inside of each foot, lengthwise, from the large toe to the heel (see illustration).

Notice in Chart C how close the bladder reflex is to the reflex of the lower lumbar region. By just moving the thumb a little bit toward the heel you will be on the reflex to the lower lumbar region and the end of the spine or tailbone.

Visual Cross-Section of Spinal Column Reflex Area

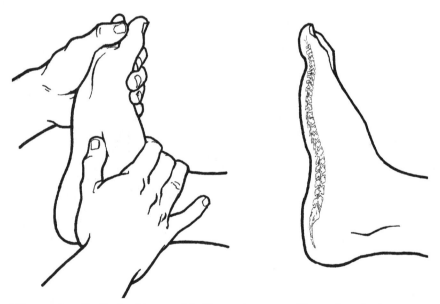

Illustration 9. By looking at this illustration you will see that the large toe represents the head and neck. The reflexes to the spine run lengthwise, from the middle of the big toe, down along the boney instep to the heel area. The reflex to the spine is found in both feet.

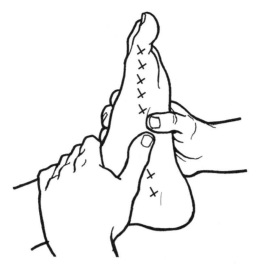

Illustration 10. Use two thumbs to stimulate both sides of the spinal reflex to aid healing circulation.

Keep this picture in mind and you will have no trouble recognizing a weakness in the back by the location of tenderness on the inside of the foot. When tenderness is found, work it gently at first, as it may be extremely tender, but know that what you are doing is causing a definite relaxing effect on the spine. If there is an injury to the spine, or if it is in any way out of alignment, you will find that as you relax the tension in the spinal reflexes, your muscles will cease to contract. Thus in nature's own way the vertebra will be able to return to its natural position, restoring once again the proper circulation.

Another method of relaxing tension around the spine is to place both thumbs on instep of foot; with a rolling-pressing motion, work up and down the foot. Press around each vertebra reflex on both feet.

Remember when working on the spinal reflexes that every part of your body receives its nerve supply from some part of the spine. An impinged nerve tightening the muscles, thus causing abnormal tension, causes most of our ailments. (See Chart H.)

Reflexes for Full Length of Spine

It is wise to work the reflexes for the full length of the spinal column for at least 2 or 3 minutes each time the feet are worked on. Thus tension on the whole spinal area is relaxed, and muscles will cease to contract. The spinal vertebrae will become realigned and circulation will be as nature intended.

THE CONNECTION BETWEEN YOUR SPINE AND NERVOUS SYSTEM

Nature chose to protect the delicate structures of the brain, spinal cord, and spinal nerves as much as possible by placing them within protective armor. Your brain is housed within the skull, and the vertebrae (backbones) are home to the spinal cord. The spinal cord runs through little holes in the vertebrae, then branches out along the spine and connects with the tissues of the body, providing them with nerve control. A study of Chart H will help you understand how important it is to protect the spinal cord. You should have a good knowledge of the spine and its relationship to the rest of the body.

CASE HISTORIES OF SPINAL HEALINGS

Following are two cases which prove beyond a doubt the therapeutic value of reflexology for the spine.

A woman went skating with her children, and had a very bad fall, landing on the end of her spine. She called me the next day to come over and see if I could bring her some relief; she had called a bone specialist to take x-rays but it would be two days before she could see him and she was in much pain. I went to her house and upon reflexing her feet found severe tenderness in the lower lumbar region, which I proceeded to work very gently. The full length of the foot on the spinal area was affected to some degree, but the lower lumbar reflex was so sensitive that I could barely touch it at first. I changed from one foot to the other often, though I found the reflex on the right foot much more tender than that on the left, indicating that she had injured the right side of the spine. After about a half hour of working the spine reflexes, the pain subsided and she was able to get up and do her work. She felt so much better that, despite my urgings for her to go to a doctor for an examination, she called the bone specialist and canceled her appointment. She took a few more reflex sessions from me, and although her back was sore for quite a while after

Nerves that regulate various parts of the body	Spinal Sections	Spine
The head and its sense organs (including a few autonomic reactions) are controlled by 12 pairs of Caranial nerves.	Brain stem	
The neck and arms are controlled by 8 pairs of Cervical nerves.	7 Vertebrae Cervical spine (neck)	
The chest cavity is regulated by 12 Thoracic nerves.	12 Vertebrae of chest area Thoracic Spine (Middle back)	
The legs and feet are manipulated by the 5 pairs of Lumbar nerves.	5 Vertebrae of lower back Lumbar Spine (lower back)	
The pelvic organs and muscles in the buttocks are managed by 6 pairs of nerves from the sacrum and coccyx.	Sacrum coccyx (Tailbone)	

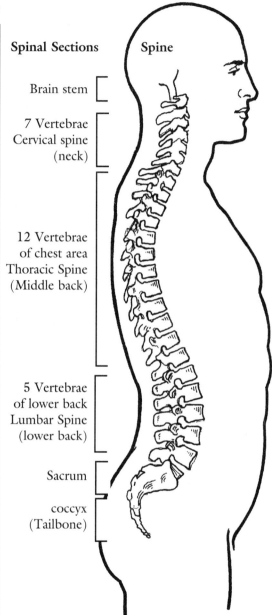

Chart H

her accident, she fully recovered. That was about ten years ago. Of course, if I had suspected any broken bones, I would have taken her immediately to the hospital.

The Author's Experience

The second case involves me. I was fishing in a small stream and as I stepped on a rock it turned with me. I quickly threw my weight onto another rock which also turned under my foot, throwing me off balance and into the stream. I landed on my back on a rock in the shallow water. The pain was so severe that I think I passed out for a second; the cold water rushing over my face revived me. I crawled out onto the bank and lay there awhile, but forced myself to get up, as I did not want to lie there long enough to become too stiff to walk. It was over a mile to the car, and I had to drive 70 miles over mountainous roads to get home.

I suffered terrible pain all night after arriving home. The next day I had to paint my living room because I was moving into a new house; every time I tried to climb the ladder to paint the ceiling I was in such pain I had to quit. I hadn't been studying reflexology very long at this time, but I knew of its benefits, so I sat down in the middle of the floor and took one of my feet in my hands.

I had struck my back about 3 inches above the waistline when I fell on the rock, so I felt along the inside of my foot up just a little from the center, and there I found a spot so tender that it made tears come to my eyes to touch it. I knew I had the right spot so I persisted with a gentle workout, first on one foot, then on the other, until I got some of the soreness worked out.

In my case, as in the previous case, most of the tenderness was in one foot. After about 20 minutes of using a press-and-roll technique, a lot of the soreness had been worked out. To my own amazement, when I got up my back was so improved that I was able to finish painting the very large room. The severe pain in my back never returned, though it was a little sore for about ten days.

There Is No Time Limit on Working Reflexes for the Back

Those of the back and other bone areas may be worked for an unlimited time, unlike those for the glands where time must be limited to a few seconds for the first few sessions. Following is a most interesting case history on a very involved situation concerning the back and related disorders.

Case History of a Serious Back Situation and Its Healing

At a dance I was introduced to a man who I thought at the time was a hunchback. I thought about the tragedy of such a nice looking man being so deformed. He stood slumped over with a big bulge standing out along his back and shoulders. I found him to be quite a good dancer and later became better acquainted with him.

I learned that he had suffered family tragedies which had made him quite despondent. I got around to telling him about the reflexology sessions I gave and how they had proved to be doing such amazing things for those who tried them. He had never heard of them before and was intensely interested. He said he had several health problems and would like to give these treatments a try.

When he arrived in my office and I had him seated comfortably in the chair, I learned that besides having a bad back he suffered from several other complaints. All of the reflexes were quite tender, and as I worked down to the stomach reflex under the area of the reflexes to the thyroid, I noticed that it was exceptionally sensitive to the touch. "Do you have stomach trouble?" I asked him. "I have an ulcer," he replied. As I worked on down the foot I found that the kidneys were also very tender. He admitted to having spells of trouble with what he had suspected were kidney problems.

As I worked the liver reflex under the little toe area on the right foot and found it very sore, I went to the reflexes of the colon and found them just as tender as the ones to the liver. I asked him if he had any trouble with constipation and his reply to that was, "I have been constipated off and on most of my life. I know you can't help that, it's just the way I am." I said, "Wait and see."

Then as my fingers moved down to the ankles, I learned that he had a lot of tenderness in the reflexes to the prostate gland. I asked him if he had known of a weakness there, but he said that he hadn't. I asked if he had to get up nights; he said that he did, several times, but often unnecessarily. So he laid the blame to nerves.

Men usually become quite upset when you mention that there might be a weakness in the prostate gland. Reflexology seems to bring new life to the prostate through added circulation and a renewal of life forces. These energy forces are able to get through and disperse the congestion that has started to build up in this gland. I have never treated a case of prostate trouble without great success.

I was able to assure my patient that his prostate condition was not serious and he would find relief within a few days. It is amazing how quickly the prostate responds when the reflexes under the ankles on the inside of the feet are worked.

As I continued to work on the feet of my patient I also found that he suffered from hay fever and sinus. The poor man had really gotten himself out of harmony with the universe, I thought, as I worked each reflex gently. He was the type that would suffer in silence and it was hard to know how hard to press without causing undue pain during the first reflex. It is unnecessary to press hard initially because the reflexes will become less tender with each session after the third, unless of course we come up against something that is chronic or cannot be helped with reflexology alone.

I knew that I was going to find quite a reaction when I started on the back reflexes, so I had left this until the last. All of the area below the big toe following the bone on the inside of the foot down to about the center of the foot was so sore that it was even more than he could stand without flinching. He told me that he had been hurt in military service, but that nothing had been done about it because it was just before they shipped out to go overseas in World War II, and so many of the boys were faking illnesses and injuries to keep from going over to fight. He said he had suffered off and on ever since, and as he grew older it became worse. At times he would be in such pain when he tried to get out of bed in the morning that he couldn't move. Sometimes he would lie in agony for as long as three weeks. He had gone to all kinds of doctors. They all agreed that he had a very bad spine but did not know what to do unless they operated on it. He was thinking seriously of resorting to that as a last hope of relief.

I tried to build up his hopes by telling him of the many cases of back troubles I had helped with reflexology.

This man suffered from both mental and physical problems that would have made many men give up all hope a long time ago. He had heavy worries and a broken heart from the loss of his family, which was in part responsible for some of his physical complaints, but not the back discomfort. His legs had started to go numb at times and he had a dead feeling in part of one leg, which he had noticed ever since he was first injured in the Navy.

After taking several reflex sessions, my patient had recovered beyond his belief. All signs of the prostate trouble vanished after the second treatment, and he said he slept all night without moving. In fact, he slept at every opportunity he had for the next month. It seemed that he just couldn't get enough sleep, he said. I told him that it was his body healing, since all of its functions had been reawakened by the life forces and a new surge of circulation throughout his whole system. His body mechanisms were literally turned loose after the reflexes were stimulated enough to allow nature to go to work as she was intended to.

It was interesting to watch the symptoms of each revealed illness disappear one by one. As his nerves grew calm and his mental depression vanished like a mist, he became more cheerful and the ulcer disappeared. He had no more kidney attacks, and for the first time that he could remember he was free of constipation and has never been bothered with it since.

Over a period of time, with regular reflex workouts, he stopped having headaches. As the muscles in the back started to relax, he was able to stand straighter every day. He was not deformed at all; he had just given the appearance of a hunchback because he was pulled forward and over by pain and tight muscles. Of course, the injured spine is still as it was, but he very seldom has any pain, and never any attacks that lay him up as they used to.

That all took place quite a few years ago and none of his old symptoms have ever returned. I know this is a fact, because I did such a good job of returning this particular man to perfect health with reflexology that I married him!

Reflexes for the Thyroid and Parathyroid

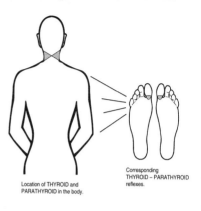

Location of THYROID and PARATHYROID in the body.

Corresponding THYROID – PARATHYROID reflexes.

We are now ready to work the reflexes to the thyroid gland, another endocrine gland and extremely important to one's well-being. Study the basic charts in the beginning of this book and glance at the illustration above to see where in the body the thyroid is located; then take a look at Photo 14 showing the position of the thyroid being reflexed.

The right foot is being held by the left hand, and the right hand is used for the reflex work. Notice how the thumb is pressed under the big toe, toward the center of the foot.

Start at the base of the big toe with the thumb pressing in the basal joint as much as possible. Work this area well. Now we will check for tenderness in the assistant, or helper, reflex of this very influential gland. Use a rolling motion and follow the bone down to the inside edge of the foot. Work along this pad covering the toe bone with the thumb or a self-help tool. If using the reflex probe, roll the sharp edge back and forth as much under the bone as possible.

Press along this pad until you hit the reflex to the thyroid. You will experience a sharp pain, and the whole area may be quite tender, with the pain very pronounced at first, but eventually the crystals will be broken loose and washed away by the released bloodstream. You will notice the pain becoming less and less.

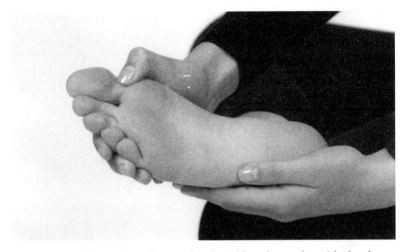

Photo 14. Working the reflex to the thyroid and parathyroid gland. Press-and-roll thumb at the base of your big toe. Also stimulate the assistant reflex areas, by working completely around the basal joint of big toe; and by moving thumb between big toe and second toe, and working down the top half of the ball of the foot.

Sometimes you will have to dig quite deeply to reach this reflex. It is especially deep on some men.

This important hormone-producing gland is not to be neglected. Often one is able to feel this crunching of accumulated crystals as pressure is applied.

THE IMPORTANCE OF THE THYROID

The thyroid is a small gland shaped like a butterfly, and is almost as light, weighing less than an ounce in most people. It is located in front of the throat, and has two lobes, one on either side of the windpipe.

The thyroid regulates the body's temperature, and releases vital hormones in the blood which influence the rate of metabolism (energy production), the rate at which food and oxygen are converted into heat and energy.

There are two hormones that regulate energy: thyroxine and tri-iodothyronine. A metabolic rate above normal can result in nervousness, emotional disturbance, loss of weight, and often feeling too warm. If the metabolic rate is low, the body will slow down in its functions, will get tired easily, will gain weight rapidly, and will feel cold.

Remember the importance of the thyroid gland when you are working its reflexes. Any derangement of this gland may affect the other glands, especially the pituitary and the adrenals. The hormones sent into the bloodstream by the thyroid gland are very important for breaking down the waste products of the body. Its malfunction can be the starting point for various problems, including profound internal changes, high blood pressure, and kidney troubles. Interestingly, many criminals and inmates of mental institutions may be victims of a thyroid deficiency.

There are substitutes for glandular hormones to temporarily provide relief, such as ACTH, cortisone, insulin, etc. However, you can restore the natural functioning of your endocrine glands by working the reflexes to each one of these glands faithfully until they have returned to normal.

If you are one of those individuals who feels as though you were born tired, finds your mentality becoming dull, feels inattentive and sleepy, you may need the hormone secretion produced by the thyroid gland to supply your body with the fuel and energy to wake you up and give you that lift that you need. Work the reflex to the thyroid, and enable it to produce its own normal secretion of the iodine-protein compound called thyroxine, helping to balance your metabolic function according to nature's plan.

REFLEXES OF THE PARATHYROIDS

If you will look again at the beginning of the book at Chart E of the endocrine glands, you will notice the location of the four tiny parathyroid glands. There are two on each side of the thyroid and are attached on the back of the lobes. They secrete a hormone which controls calcium in the blood.

You can easily see that you will use the same position and the same location to work these tiny but very significant glands. You will have to press in a little deeper than you do for the thyroid. Generally, the parathyroids will get enough benefit from working the thyroid reflex, unless there is a definite congestion within them.

This also is the gland that is responsible for your poise and tranquility, besides many other important body functions which I will explain further in Chapter 25.

The probe will probably be needed to reach these reflexes in order to press back in behind the thyroid reflexes. Be very careful not to bruise the tissue or capillaries with the deep pressure.

When you get through working the reflexes to the thyroid and parathyroid glands on the one foot, change positions and work the opposite foot in the same manner.

Reflex Areas to the Lungs and Bronchial Tubes

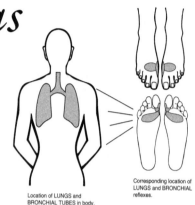

Location of LUNGS and BRONCHIAL TUBES in body.

Corresponding location of LUNGS and BRONCHIAL reflexes.

Let's look again at Charts A and B to see the position of the lungs. Notice how they lie in the chest, and then note how the reflexes to the lungs are situated along the pads of the feet which lie below the toes, under the reflexes to the eyes and the ears. You will also notice that the lungs take up quite a large space in the chest area. Similarly the reflexes to the lungs take up quite an area on the foot. Remember, right foot, right lung; left foot, left lung.

Hold the right foot with the left hand and use the fingers of the right hand to work along the reflexes to the lungs. Use a circular, rolling motion as you cover the whole pad under the toes. Use of the probe will make the reflex work of this area easier, by rolling it across the foot, back and forth, and also up and down, so that the whole area may be well covered.

You can also work diagonally in a criss-crossing technique to cover this large area of reflexes. To do this, thumb-walk in a diagonal direction from the diaphragm reflex up to the toes; make several trips, starting at one edge of the foot and work your way across the other edge. Change hands. With opposite thumb, work over the same area; however, this time you will be traveling across the foot in the other direction (see Illustration 26 on page 249).

If your fingers are sore or tired, use your probe for the criss-cross technique.

The trachea (windpipe) and lungs are part of the respiratory system which delivers oxygen to the blood. The lungs consist of millions of elastic membranous sacs which together can hold about as much air as a basketball. They are constantly inflating and emptying in their crucial capacity as a medium of exchange.

The lungs sustain life by unloading carbon dioxide and taking in oxygen carried by the blood to the cells. Oxygen unlocks the energy contained in the body's fuels. The body's trillions of cells require so much oxygen that we need about 30 times as much surface for its intake as our entire skin area covers. The lungs provide this surface area (even though they weigh only about 2½ pounds on the average, and fit neatly within the chest cavity). This is due to the fact that their membranes fold over and over on themselves in pockets thinner than a sheet of paper, so thin that gases pass right through them. The lungs trade air with blood. As the heart pumps old blood to the lungs, they relieve the blood of unnecessary waste products and carbon dioxide. Then they give fresh oxygen to the blood and return it to the heart to repeat the cycle.

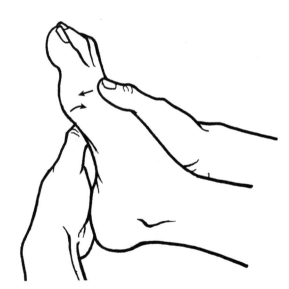

Illustration 11. Using both thumbs, work the lung and bronchial reflex area; press and roll thumbs simultaneously.

Even the purest country air contains dust particles and bacteria. City air, of course, is additionally burdened with soot and exhaust fumes. As the air passes through the nose, some of its dust particles and bacteria drop off; others are trapped by tiny hairs or mucus. In the windpipe, most of the remaining bacteria in the air are intercepted by mucus.

Since the respiratory system is of major importance to good health, let's try another way to reach the reflexes. Reposition your hands so that fingers are overlapping to one side of foot, and both thumbs are free to "work the reflexes." Place one thumb on top of foot, and the other on the sole of foot. Work the reflexes with a double press-and-roll technique (using two thumbs at once) from the base of big toe (throat reflex) down to the diaphragm reflex, continuing across the foot to cover both lung and bronchial reflex areas. Always reflex both feet. (See illustration 11.)

BRONCHIAL TUBES

The bronchi are two large tubes, one passage way for each lung, leading off the trachea (or windpipe) like the limbs of a tree. They then taper on down into smaller bronchi tubes to make a treelike formation within the lungs. You can see how disastrous it is for the body when a severe infection of these muscular bronchi results in destruction of the muscle necessary for contraction.

Reflexing the whole area of the lungs will benefit the bronchial tubes. Hold the same position as when working the lung reflexes. Start applying pressure under the big toe, in the same place as the throat reflexes, so that you will be sure to cover the reflexes to the larynx (or vocal cords) at the top of the trachea (windpipe).

With your thumb, press into the soft area starting under the big toe and walk your thumb down to the pad under the toes. If there is any tenderness, concentrate on it with a pressing, circular motion. If there is any indication of congestion in the lungs or the bronchials, then make sure you work all reflexes of the respiratory system (which includes the nose, throat, larynx, trachea, bronchi, and lungs). Cover these areas thoroughly. If you do not find tenderness, you may not be getting deep enough. We know that where there is congestion there is trouble, so work it out.

COLDS

While we are on the subject of the lungs, I want to mention the effects of colds. A cold is nature's way of cleaning house, that is, eliminating the system of toxic acid. It is trying to rid the body of accumulated poisons, through the pores of the skin and the mucous membrane in the head, nose, and sinuses. So do not work the reflexes to the whole body when you have a cold. Remember, it is already overburdened with eliminating poisons, so just give nature a little help instead of hindrance by working the toes and chest-lung reflex area. Include a very *short* workout of the kidney reflex. The pituitary reflex can be concentrated on in case of fever.

CHAPTER 10

How to Handle Stomach Reflexes

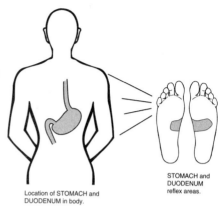

Location of STOMACH and DUODENUM in body.

STOMACH and DUODENUM reflex areas.

The stomach lies high in the abdomen, on the left side, nested up under the diaphragm and protected by the rib cage. In form it is kind of a pouch, about 10 inches long, with a diameter that depends on its contents. When full, it can stretch to hold as much as 2 quarts of food. When empty, it collapses on itself like a deflated balloon. Food materials take the same route along the gastrointestinal tract, whether slated to be converted into energy or to be eliminated as waste. Food's entry into the stomach—as well as its exit therefrom—is regulated by circular muscles which act somewhat like purse strings, alternately expanding and contracting. The stomach works on the food both mechanically and chemically. The movement of the stomach walls mashes the food, kneading it as a cook kneads dough. This permits the thorough mixing in of a digestive juice, the chief ingredients of which are pepsin and hydrochloric acid.

The stomach's principal role is to mix digestive juices from small glands that dissolve and break foods down into semifluids. The strong stomach walls have muscles that crush, stir, and mash foods for about three hours, then push the thick liquid paste easily into the small intestine.

Study Chart A a moment; notice that it shows the stomach positioned almost in the center of the body, although in reality the stomach lies mostly on the left side. However, it is made of muscle and can

88

stretch to the size of a big balloon. We find the reflexes to be a bit more on the left foot, but work on both feet. These charts are not drawn for anatomical accuracy, but rather to make it convenient for the layman to find the reflexes in relation to certain parts of the body.

Now look at Photo 15 and notice the position of using the knuckle of the forefinger.

This is a handy position to use on some of the reflexes. By using the knuckle you can exert more pressure in some areas, and it doesn't seem to get as tired as the thumb. If you don't have a reflex probe or some kind of similar self-help tool, then alternating the thumb and the knuckle works satisfactorily.

Let's start reflexing. Since you have some idea of the workings of the stomach, you can now understand how much benefit you can give this all-important organ by stimulating it with reflexology.

STOMACH REFLEX TECHNIQUES

Take the left foot up into position; bend the finger of the right hand and press the knuckle into the reflexes of the stomach as shown in Photo 15. Press with the same rolling motion that you use with the thumb. Work from the center of the foot toward the inside, clear to the spine reflexes. Press in and up under the pad as much as possible. Feel those tender buttons in there? You will probably find it especial-

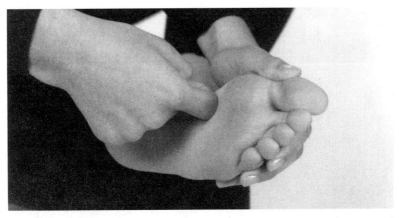

Photo 15. Using the knuckle to stimulate healing energy to the stomach, solar plexus, and diaphragm.

ly tender just as you reach the spine reflex below the bronchial reflexes. This may be more sensitive on the left foot because the stomach pouch is more on the left side of the body.

Does it hurt? Some of these reflexes are so tender and hurt so badly that tears will come to your eyes, or you may have to grit your teeth as you reflex. But your instinct will demand that you keep on rubbing. It is nature's call for new life, which at last you have learned how to give, in a harmless, rejuvenating way. You can reflex very gently at first, increasing the pressure as the tenderness diminishes, and it will, in a surprisingly short time. Some reflexes will recover faster than others.

Remember the job your stomach has to do for you. To enjoy perfect health, always chew your food well before swallowing it; otherwise, foods that have not been chewed well can cause the muscles to relax and contract in such a fast rhythmic movement that you will get a stomach ache. Help make your stomach's job a little easier; it will reward you—by not hurting.

HOW TO SOOTHE AWAY ULCERS

Ulcers are very common, afflicting between 10 and 15 percent of the population. Much mystery still surrounds their origin. No one seems to know why they occur more frequently in men than in women.

Peptic ulcers commonly erupt within the digestive system. These open sores often surface in the stomach, esophagus, or duodenum (which is the first ten inches of the small intestine).

Research has shown that some ulcers result from a malfunction of the pituitary and adrenal glands. Here again we have the related action of the glands. I hope you are beginning to understand how reflexology can bring your body back to complete health. In giving yourself these treatments, you are not only treating one malfunction that you think is causing your illness but all parts of the body, so that you are sure of getting every organ and gland back in harmony with each other.

Not only emotions cause ulcers, nor do they solely afflict the digestive system. Nevertheless, the influence of emotions is evident in a host of ailments, ranging all the way from skin irritations, such as hives and eczema, to fatal heart attacks.

The relationship between emotions and digestion has been known for centuries: the dry mouth or empty sensation at the pit of the stomach caused by fear; the heavy stomach that accompanies depression; or the cramping pain of tension. No wonder ulcers soon heal when treated with reflexology. Both the body and the mind are bathed in a soothing, relaxing sensation.

If you think you have ulcers, you will work not only the reflexes to the stomach, but also the pituitary and adrenals to relax the emotions. Many people have recovered completely from ulcers through reflexology.

It is said that a dog does not have ulcers, as he will go off in a dark corner and completely relax when he feels badly, and an ulcer has no power then to progress from bad to worse.

When we talk of the stomach we think of food. Do you consider your stomach when you are eating?

Case Histories of Ulcer Pain Disappearing

Mr. H. had mistreated his system so badly that he actually became allergic to food of every kind. Doctors told him there was nothing they could do for him, and in desperation he turned to reflexology as a last resort. Now, several years later, he maintains his perfect health.

Mr. L. was bringing a load of horses to California from New Mexico. He became very ill on the way, with bad stomach pains. He said he had been having trouble with his stomach for the past few months but had not done anything about it. Now he knew he would have to stop and see a doctor, but what to do with the truckload of horses? As he drove along the highway he saw a sign reading "Reflexology." He wasn't sure it would help but he stopped and went in. He was given a reflex treatment, and to his surprise and wonder, his stomach pains stopped during the reflexology session, and now several years later, he writes to tell us the pain still has not returned.

CHAPTER 11

How to Work the Solar Plexus and Diaphragm Reflexes

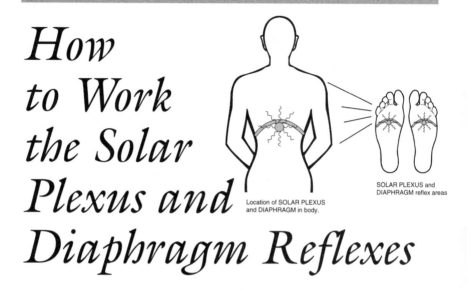

Location of SOLAR PLEXUS and DIAPHRAGM in body.

SOLAR PLEXUS and DIAPHRAGM reflex areas

The solar plexus is a network of nerve fibers situated behind the stomach and in front of the diaphragm. So when we work the stomach reflexes, we are bound to stimulate these two reflexes as well. This great network of nerves goes out to all parts of the abdominal cavity, and is sometimes called the abdominal brain. The fine interlacing of nerves extends from part of the aorta to the diaphragm, and includes the front of the abdominal aorta, as well as the adrenal glands.

The diaphragm reflex is centered in the upper middle part of each foot. The solar plexus reflex is behind that of the stomach; thus a deeper pressure is required to relax nerve impulses.

Here we will give you a few different techniques of working this important reflex area. You only need to use one technique per session. Choose the method that is easiest and most beneficial for you.

CIRCULAR-PRESS TECHNIQUE

To reflex the diaphragm and solar plexus, take the same position as for the stomach reflex. Notice in Photo 15, page 89, in the illustration for stomach reflexes, how the knuckle is located on the foot. You may find it easier to use the thumb on this reflex. One easy routine is to place your thumb on the reflex button and move it slowly in small circular motions, to the left and then to the right.

PUSH-AND-RELEASE TECHNIQUE ON SOLAR PLEXUS REFLEX

Another very effective method is the slow push-and-release motion. You can relax your whole body by reflexing this area, and taking a few deep breaths at the same time. Move the right foot into position. Now place the thumb of your right or left hand on the solar plexus reflex in the center of the foot. (Of course you remember this network of nerves includes the abdominal aorta and the adrenal glands. This is why the most powerful and effective reflex point to the solar plexus is located just above the adrenal glands in the abdominal area.)

As you gradually press deeply on the solar plexus button, also take a deep breath slowly into your lungs. Hold both your thumb and your breath for about seven seconds. Then gradually release the pressure of your thumb and your breath at the same time. Repeat this exercise five or six times, then change to the left foot and repeat.

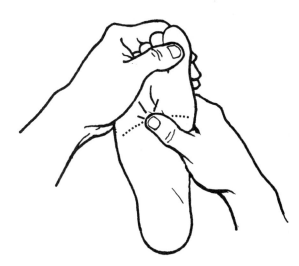

Illustration 12. Push-and-release on the solar plexus button.

WORKING THE DIAPHRAGM REFLEX

It is impossible to work the reflex to the solar plexus without affecting that of the diaphragm, which is an arching muscular wall separating the thorax (chest cavity) from the abdomen. When you inhale air into your lungs, this muscle is drawn downward, allowing the air capacity in the lungs to increase. (See Chart B.) Between the lung and stomach reflex is the diaphragm reflex.

Every time a muscle contracts, it squeezes the blood vessels, especially the veins. It is obvious how the circulatory system is benefited by reflexology.

"THUMB WALKING" THE SOLAR PLEXUS AND THE DIAPHRAGM REFLEXES

To reflex the diaphragm and solar plexus at the same time, overlap fingers on top of foot, just above the waistline. Place both of your thumbs on the sole of your foot. Using a small "walking" motion, work one thumb at a time across the diaphragm reflex area. Start with your left thumb, and "walk" it across the foot . . . then alternate and

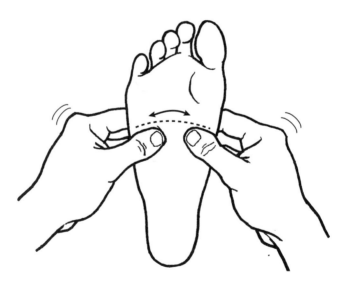

Illustration 13. Double the benefit by thumb-walking in each direction, alternating pressure with thumbs.

thumb-walk the right thumb back again. Work from one side of the foot to the other, covering both the diaphragm and solar plexus reflexes.

Working over the zones of these two valuable nerve and muscle focal points will promote a soothing and pleasurable feeling. Relaxation of this area reduces stress effectively, improves sleep, helps ease digestion, and relieves abdominal pain. Now you can use reflexology as a skillful way to successfully reduce tension in this important nerve center of your body. And don't forget to breathe healing energy into your lungs for added benefits.

CHAPTER 12

Reflexes to Adrenal Glands and Kidneys

Location of ADRENAL GLANDS and KIDNEYS in the body.

ADRENAL GLAND and KIDNEY reflex areas.

You have a kidney and adrenal on each side of the body, so you will have a kidney and adrenal reflex on each foot. Let's look at Photo 16 and notice the position for working the reflex to the adrenal and kidney. In this illustration of the Reflex Roller in use, the roller is pressed vertically into the foot, almost in the center, just above the reflex for the colon and just below the diaphragm reflex.

Take the right leg and get into position so you can easily reach the foot with the left hand. You may use your thumb, a self-help tool such as the Reflex Roller, the Hand Probe, or another similar tool, as long as you are able to press in deeply enough to reach the reflex buttons under the skin.

The adrenal fits on top of the kidney like a little hat, so when you reflex the kidney, you will also be reflexing the adrenal, especially if you are using one of the helpful reflex devices. The kidney reflex lies vertically on the foot, with the adrenal reflex up toward the toes. You can see that the Reflex Roller (also known as Rollo-Reflex-Massager) will cover larger areas of the reflexes, more than just the thumb or the little Hand Probe. (The Probe is more convenient to use when trying to find a pinpointed spot, or when testing for tenderness before reflexing. It is also excellent for working small areas such as the toes, between the toes, and areas with thick skin such as the heels.)

When using the Reflex Roller to stimulate renewed energy in the pathways to the adrenals and kidneys, roll it up and down, along zones 3, 2, and 1. Look at Charts A and B. See how the adrenals and kidneys are located in zones 3 and 2. The urethra, which is a passage tube that carries urine to the bladder, crosses over the zones and down to the bladder in zone 1.

Visualize how the urinary system works. Then reflex from the adrenal gland down to the kidney. Continue on down the urethra and into the bladder reflex. Follow the flow of the urinary system as you reflex. See Illustration 14 on page 99 of this chapter. You will be sending vital energy to help flush out the waste gathered from the blood in the kidney, through the urethra, down into the bladder. When full, the bladder will then eliminate the waste and urine from the body.

SPECIAL TECHNIQUE FOR ACTIVATING THE ADRENAL GLANDS

With the right foot in place, supported with the right hand, place your left thumb in a vertical position in the center of the foot, just on

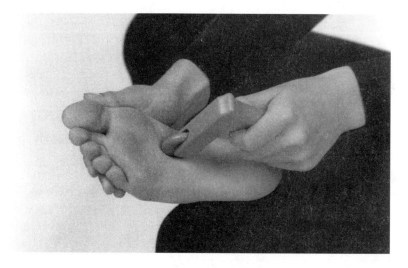

Photo 16. The Reflexer Roller is a wonderful self-help tool, designed to help reach the reflex areas with ease. It is especially beneficial to those who have arthritic fingers, or tired, sore hands. This position shows the Rollo stimulating the reflex area to the kidney and adrenal gland.

top of the kidney reflex. Now move the thumb up just a little toward the toes. Press in with the tip of your thumb (down a bit from the solar plexus reflex). Press in with a downward pull. Always be gentle at first, then work to a firmer pressure.

The two adrenal glands are critical to the body's natural functions. They help maintain fluid balance and are important to reproduction. Adrenals also produce adrenalin for the body when it needs extra energy in the case of an emergency.

The action of the adrenal is often influenced by fright, anger, and many kinds of distress. So if you feel this might be the cause of an abnormally functioning adrenal, it would serve well to give special attention to the solar plexus, which is a network of nerve fibers. Test it for soreness; if it is tender, press and hold the reflex for a few seconds. (Refer to Illustration 12, on page 93.)

The adrenal glands are part of the endocrine system. Look at Chart E of the endocrine glands, and keep in mind that if the reflex to any one of these glands is tender, then the others are almost sure to show some degree of tenderness as well.

Remember that the pituitary hormones influence other organs and glands, to keep them functioning correctly. They even control the amount of urine the kidneys make. The adrenal gland produces 30 or more steroid hormones, and is especially influenced by a certain substance produced by the pituitary. Always double check the pituitary reflex for soreness when there is trouble with the adrenals. All endocrine glands must be balanced so that the body can function properly.

SPECIAL TECHNIQUE FOR REFLEXING THE KIDNEYS

With the thumb still in the same position as working the adrenal, use a rolling-pressing motion on the reflex, just below the adrenals. Work on down to the colon reflex below the waistline, and this will stimulate the kidney reflex.

Another helpful technique is to place your thumb on the kidney reflex point, and with the opposite hand, rotate the top of the foot to the left, then to the right. You may want to use this technique during your next reflex session, as you do not want to overstimulate the kidney reflexes the first few times. As you may recall, too much toxic wastes draining from the system all at once could make you feel ill.

Each kidney is about the size of a bar of face soap, and shaped like a large kidney bean. Interestingly enough, the kidney reflex area on the bottom of your foot is about the same size as a kidney bean. The kidneys have a major job to do: they recycle liquids and regulate salt and nutrients. All the body's blood goes through the kidneys which filter and purify blood and produce urine which flushes out the wastes.

So be careful, particularly if this reflex is extremely tender. Remember that as a result of this reflexology workout, your kidneys are working hard to get rid of all the accumulated poisons and impurities that your body is now triumphantly flushing out.

HOW THE KIDNEYS AFFECT VARIOUS PORTIONS OF THE BODY

In review, the kidneys regulate salts and water balance in the blood and flush out toxins as well. Reflexology has been successful in alleviating many kidney disorders, including water retention and swelling, weakness when trying to hold urine, even bedwetting. Many times you will find the kidney reflex on one foot very tender,

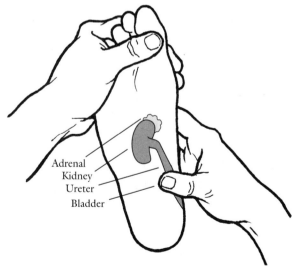

Adrenal
Kidney
Ureter
Bladder

Illustration 14. Working reflex area of the urinary tract.

while that to the other kidney on the opposite foot will show very little or no tenderness at all. Definitely the one showing the tender reflex is not contracting and relaxing as nature intended, and is thus allowing congestion to form. It does not make any difference when doing reflexology if the kidneys are overactive, causing too frequent urination, or if they are underactive. Reflexology will correct and restore the kidney action to normal balance in a short time.

Remember that the eyes may also be affected by faulty kidneys. In case of eye trouble or weakness, don't forget the kidney reflexes as well as those to the eyes and neck.

Nature's tendency is to restore all the body's systems to normal conditions when we give her back the necessary circulation, so that she can rebuild the sick and broken-down glands and organs of the body.

Reducing the Risk of Stones

While we are working on the kidney reflex, we will mention kidney stones from which it is said one out of five people suffer. In treating this condition with reflexology, concentrate on relaxing the whole urinary tract. Remember to work between the kidney and the bladder, back and forth on the ureter reflex, relaxing the tension so nature can eliminate the kidney stones through normal muscular contraction.

In Chapter 8, we learned that the parathyroids regulate calcium absorption. For this reason it is very important to work the parathyroid reflex if you suspect a urinary or kidney stone problem. Overactive parathyroids allow increased mineral absorption into the body which can solidify into stones.

A Preventive Diet Is Important

It is significantly important to watch your diet to reduce the risk of stones. Cut back on high fat and high animal protein foods to reduce the risk of uric acid and waste buildup. Limit foods rich in calcium, such as real butter, cheese, whole milk, and other dairy products. Some foods should be avoided if at all possible, such as spinach, swiss chard, chocolate, and tomatoes, because they are high in the acid that forms calcium oxalates, the material ordinarily found in stones.

It is essential to drink lots of good water; a full glass every hour would benefit the urinary system. Raw foods and fresh juices, especially cranberry juice, and raw unpasteurized apple cider vinegar (1 T. to 6-oz. glass of water) help acidify the urine and kill bacteria. Our family has found that the herb K-B is a wonderful diuretic; it can be found wherever vitamins are sold.

It is immensely important to have your urinary system in complete balance. So make certain to treat your kidneys kindly, and give them some reflex-stimulation. However, don't overdo, as working too long can cause a feeling of discomfort.

Your body wants to be healthy, which it will be by continuously flushing itself of detrimental waste. Give it the help it needs, and at the same time regain your natural good health and celebrate renewed vitality.

CHAPTER 13

Reflexes to Pancreas and Spleen

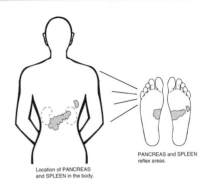

Location of PANCREAS and SPLEEN in the body.

PANCREAS and SPLEEN reflex areas.

While we are learning to reflex the kidney and adrenals, let us look once more at Chart E of the endocrine glands. Notice how the pancreas lies horizontally between the kidneys. The reflex for the pancreas lies in a band extending nearly all the way across the left foot, and nearly halfway across the right foot.

A SPECIAL REFLEX TECHNIQUE

To work the reflex to the pancreas gland you will take the same position as for working the kidneys. Study the chart and the illustrations; see how this gland runs across the body instead of up and down as the kidneys do. So work across the foot, between the instep to the kidney reflexes. Work clear across the left foot and halfway across the right foot, if you are centralizing your attention on this particular gland.

But, as we have observed, the reflexes to this gland lie in about the same place as other glands and organs within the abdominal cavity. The pancreas is located below, as well as behind, the stomach. It is generally stimulated when you work the reflexes in this area of the foot; therefore this gland needs little special attention. If there appears to be tenderness in any area of the pancreas, work it out.

Many of these glands lie one behind the other in the body, so the reflexes will be confined to a small area on the feet. It is sensible not to try too hard to decide which button goes to which gland, but merely follow the rule: *When there is tenderness, work it out.*

The pancreas gland must be treated respectfully as one of the major balancing mechanisms of your metabolism. This is the maker of insulin, a hormone which lowers the sugar in the bloodstream.

Actually the pancreas has several jobs to do, and functions as both an endocrine gland and an exocrine organ. The endocrine section of the pancreas sends out hormones directly into the bloodstream. Among these hormones are insulin and glucagon, which are both important substances to help the body convert sugars into energy, and keep the correct level of sugar in the bloodstream. The exocrine section of the pancreas produces special chemicals called enzymes, which break down the starches, sugars, and fats in the digestive system.

WARNING FOR DIABETICS

So here is a *warning* to those who have *diabetes*: remember to keep track of your insulin level, especially when using reflexology. During this process, you may induce a normal increase in the supply of insulin. Since the pancreas regulates the production of insulin, the reflex-stimulation of this gland may affect the insulin level.

Over the years I have had many patients who returned to me after a few sessions with the news that their doctors reduced their insulin, or discontinued their prescriptions of insulin completely.

Keep in mind that insulin shots or patches are not a cure, as they do not induce the pancreas to work better, nor do they help the pancreas return to normal.

There are so many people who do not know that they have diabetes, yet feel they are living only half a life. Many times grief or shock will affect the entire glandular system and the result will be diabetes. This type of diabetes will usually respond to reflexology and not require so many treatments as will a longstanding case.

Diabetes in children is sometimes caused by a virus; other times their immune system destroys the insulin-producing cells. Doctors tell us there is no cure for these children. However, we know that reflexology cannot hurt; it only benefits Nature in her attempt to heal the body by granting a normal circulatory system. I would say have faith and reflex anyway. I have seen some marvelous things happen, that surprised me many times, when doctors had said it couldn't be done.

Don't forget to look for tenderness in other gland reflexes, especially the thyroid glands and the pituitary.

Also search for sore spots in the liver reflex area, to balance the sugar level. The liver works with the pancreas; it is a reserve for extra sugar. When the pancreas produces the hormone glucagon, it stimulates the liver to release sugar into the blood, thus raising the blood sugar levels as needed.

If you are a diabetic, you must educate your family and friends to the symptoms and what action they should take if you show any signs of a problem.

THE SPLEEN

The spleen serves as a storehouse for iron needed by the blood. It is a fragile sponge-like organ, with a thin covering; yet it is very versatile. The spleen filters out harmful bacteria and damaging elements from the blood. It also removes particles of broken-down red cells from the blood.

The spleen helps produce disease-fighting white blood cells, and serves as a reserve for additional blood.

Reflex of the Spleen

Turn back to Chart A, and look at the spleen. See how it is located on the left side of the body. It lies behind the far left side of the stomach, and is protected by the ribs. The reflex button to the spleen is in about the same position on the left foot as the gallbladder reflex button on the right foot, except that it is slightly closer to the outer edge of the foot.

You have just finished reflexing the pancreas. While still holding the left foot, place your thumb at the end of the pancreas reflex and move it toward the outside edge and upward a bit; here you will find the spleen reflex. This will be a small area in which to work, and since it lies under the reflex area for the heart and arteries, it will generally get its share of stimulation when you are working the heart and circulatory reflexes.

Anemic Conditions

If you find that the reflex area for the spleen has any tenderness at all, then you may be somewhat anemic. Improvement can be so rapid it is amazing. With pernicious anemia, results will be slower, but nature will be there, changing new blood cells for old.

Cause of Anemia

Anemia is a deficiency in the amount of red blood cells, or the number of hemoglobin they hold. It is often caused by lack of iron in the blood and can create serious trouble if neglected for a long period of time. Women are more prone to be anemic than men. When I was very young I became very anemic but didn't have any idea what my trouble was. I just didn't seem to have the energy to climb out of bed, let alone walk around. The doctor said that because I was so anemic, I had the energy of a 90-year-old woman. Do you ever feel like that? Press the spleen reflex to see if you can find tenderness. If there is, then you have congestion and the spleen is not working properly. So work it out.

One day while walking down the street, I started having pains below the little toe. The pains kept bothering me, so I stooped down as if to fix my shoe, slipped my shoe off, and gave the spot a few quick digs with my finger. The pains stopped. When I got home, I sat down, picked up my left foot, and pressed around to make sure of where the warning pains had come from. I found the spot very quickly on the reflex to the spleen. Then I realized that I must be anemic again, so I reflexed the area thoroughly until most of the tenderness was gone.

A little later I accidentally cut my finger and I could see that my blood was not the rich, dark red that it should have been. Thus warned, I concentrated on iron-rich foods, a vitamin supplement with folic acid, vitamin B_{12}, an iron tonic, and, of course, reflexology to the spleen.

CHAPTER 14

How
to Reflex
the
Remarkable Liver

LIVER reflex area.

Location of
LIVER in body.

By now you have learned the correct techniques for contacting the various reflex buttons in the feet as far as we have gone. We have been working on the reflexes which have included both feet; now we come to the liver reflex, which is located only on the right foot, as you will see by looking at Chart B and the above illustration.

THE LIVER WILL REGENERATE ITSELF

The liver is part of your digestive system. Among other duties it modifies foods, produces proteins, and secretes bile. It is of vital importance, and extremely beneficial to the health and energy of your body. Without the liver's functions, death will occur. The liver is the "giver of life" (live).

The liver is the largest internal organ in the body, weighing about three pounds in an adult, and is said to perform about 500 different functions. Most of its cells are alike; therefore, if it becomes damaged, it will replace itself by regrowing new cells. But unfortunately, if the complete liver is consumed by disease, a transplant is necessary.

The liver performs many tasks. It is a natural antiseptic and purgative, and helps to supply some of the substances for bloodmaking. Perhaps it is best known for being such a great filter. It has circulating through it at all times about one-quarter of all the blood in the body. It filters out toxins and removes wastes. It even filters out alcohol in small amounts and harmful drugs, then flushes them through the kidneys.

The liver is also known as a storage house, safekeeping a variety of vitamins, minerals, and sugar until they are needed by the body.

In addition to hundreds of other activities, it plays a very important role in the digestive system by processing food and turning it into life-preserving substances. It manufactures bile to digest fats and prevent constipation, forming about two pints of bile a day. This goes into the intestines, serving as a lubricant to help avoid difficult or irregular bowel movements.

The liver is located primarily on the right side of the body. In the upper abdominal area, there is a small lobe that crosses over to the stomach, on the left side of the body.

Reflex Area of the Liver

Take your right foot and get into position for reflexing. Notice in Photo 17 how the thumb of the left hand is pressing under the pad on the outside of the foot. This is the area of the liver reflexes. Work this area with a rolling, pressing motion.

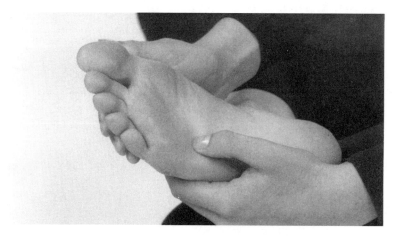

Photo 17. Working the reflex area to the remarkable liver.

Since the liver is such a large organ to cover, the reflex area consists of several buttons to contact. However, some of this area has already been stimulated when you reflexed other glands in the upper abdominal region, such as the solar plexus. And keep in mind that you do not want to overwork the kidney reflex, also found in this region.

If you are having trouble with your liver for one reason or another, and find soreness in this reflex area, you may want to work clear across the right foot, from zone 5 to zone 1 and back again. Use your press-and-roll or a criss-cross technique. Start at the outside of the foot and work toward the spine reflex. Then change hands and reflex from the spine reflex back toward the outside of the foot. This will cover the entire reflex area to the liver.

If you find tenderness in this area, indicating a sluggish liver, it will be more in the nature of a dull pain, rather than the sharp pains characterizing other reflexes you have previously worked. You will then know that the liver is sluggish and lacks the proper circulation and muscular action to function properly. When the normal function of this important gland has been neglected over a long period of time, it can result in diabetes, gallstones, jaundice, atrophy, sclerosis, constipation, etc. There is no doubt of the wonderful healing results you can

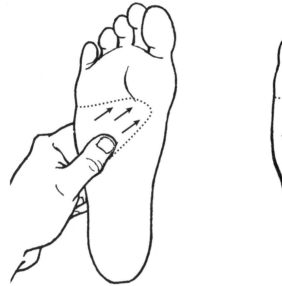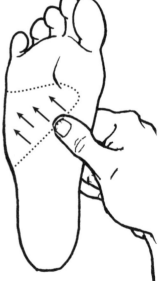

Illustration 15.   Criss-crossing the liver reflex area on the right foot.

obtain by working the reflex area of the liver. So continue using a firm pressure, so that the natural circulation can be restored, lessening any obstructions to good health.

WARNING ABOUT A SLUGGISH LIVER

Let me warn you about a very sluggish liver, which would have a very sensitive reflex when touched. Work it very lightly, and for only a few seconds the first time. You can expect several different reactions from this treatment for the liver. In severe cases it is best not to work these reflexes again for several days. Give nature a chance to throw off excess poison and adjust itself to increased circulation which you have put in motion by working these reflexes.

Some people have felt very relieved after the first reflex session, and then when they took the second session of the liver reflexes, became quite ill as nature went to work eliminating the excess poisons released by the congested liver. After the third session taken several days later, they always felt much better and continued to show a lot of improvement with each session thereafter.

I have had patients who have had 10 and 12 bowel movements in one day after the second or third treatment. The stools at this time may be of heavy mucus, black, green, or other off-colors. This is nature doing her long-delayed house cleaning. During this time you may have a tired, listless feeling. Don't worry; think how well you will feel when nature has completed her cleaning job.

Reflex this pad under the little toe on the right foot and feel for any tenderness in the area. If the liver is enlarged, a larger area of the foot will be involved. Remember our motto, "If it hurts, reflex it."

HOW TO COPE WITH GALLBLADDER CONDITIONS

While you have the right foot in this position, let's work the reflexes to the gallbladder. Notice on Chart B how the gallbladder is just a little below and toward the center of the liver reflex. This gallbladder is lodged on the undersurface of the right lobe of the liver, and is a pear-shaped, fibro-muscular receptacle for the bile. This is also the receptacle where the very painful, hardened masses called gallstones are found. There are many cases where reflexing of the liver and gallbladder have saved people from having an operation, since the stones seemed to vanish after a few sessions. It is not known whether these stones dissolved and were flushed out, or if the sessions so relaxed the gall duct that they were passed off.

If you find any tenderness in this area at all, reflex it with either the thumb or your hand-held probe, until every bit of tenderness is gone. Don't try to rub it all out the first time, though. It took a long time to get this way, so give nature a chance to relieve this congestion, which you will know has taken place when the tenderness is no longer there.

CASE HISTORY OF CHRONIC FATIGUE OVERCOME

Jim was a big, handsome man over 6 feet tall, with a large frame. His wife was about 4 feet, 6 inches tall and had worked hard all her life supporting him and the children. He had always been too sick to work, I was told by his relatives who had recommended him to me. Just plain lazy was the only disease that Jim had, they said in disgust. I could see why they felt this way by looking at the two.

No person is just plain lazy, I told them. Everyone wants to feel full of vitality. No one is happy just lying around; it is against nature. A so-called "lazy" person is really sick. Somewhere in his body there is congestion of glands or organs that is cutting off a healthy circulation of the very life forces that keep him alive. Never condemn a lazy person; he is to be pitied.

Lazy people lie around without any show of energy and they certainly are not filled with a zest for life. They don't want to work, but they don't play either. Life is very empty. And they readily agree that they are lazy, just as heavy people will agree that they are overweight. *Lazy* should have another synonym denoting lack of energy, as other health problems have. Reflexology can help reclaim their true energy, thus improving their health and life.

Jim came to me for treatments several weeks and didn't show the improvement that I thought he should. He did have several glands that were not functioning properly, according to my findings in the reflexes of his feet; thus the feet were very tender in some places. But Jim was a baby where pain was concerned. He wiggled and twisted and moaned every time that I barely touched a tender spot any place on his feet. So I did work very gently. In fact, I didn't feel that I was doing him much good because I could not break up the crystals in the capillaries so that they could free the bloodstream of the congestion or stopped-up lines that were slowing a free flow of healing blood to his depleted glands and organs. Also I could not exert enough pressure to send the electrical life force surging through his body to recharge his vitality enough to build up his energy.

One day after I had him seated in the chair with his shoes and socks removed, I said, "Jim, you are not improving as you should, and it is because I have been too easy on you. Today I am going to give you a good working over and get something stirred up in there. Can you take it?" He said he could.

I dug in, starting with the pituitary reflex in the center of his big toe. That had improved considerably during the time he had been coming, even though I had not worked it very heavily. The thyroid had improved somewhat, too. As I went over each reflex I pressed quite deeply, and he sat there and hung onto the chair arms, gritting his teeth. Then I came to the liver reflex, my fingers pressing into the spongy area under the little toe on the right side. I thought I had lost both arms of my chair for sure. A congested, sluggish liver. What could make a person more tired than a malfunctioning liver? No wonder the poor man was called lazy all of his life. He wasn't lazy; he was sick, not enough to be sick in bed or complain about it, but he had a reason for his chronic fatigue.

Of course, the adrenals and the thyroid had a place in this lack of energy, too. Since the whole mechanism of the body had been out of balance for probably most of his existence because of the glands that did not function as they should, Jim had not lived a very pleasant life. I don't suppose he enjoyed seeing his little wife get out and support him and the children for most of their married years. But if you are so tired that it is an effort to stoop down to pick up the paper, is it fair for us more fortunate people to call you lazy?

From then on, Jim improved very rapidly and the tender spots in the bottoms of his feet vanished almost completely.

So remember to look to the reflexes of the liver to alleviate any feeling of chronic sluggishness and lack of energy. Check the adrenals and thyroid also for any sign of tenderness.

Conditioning Reflexes for the Heart

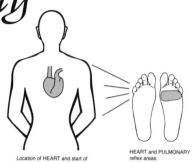

Location of HEART and start of AORTA and PULMONARY ARTERY in body.

HEART and PULMONARY reflex areas.

There probably would be no argument over the fact that the heart is one of the most important organs in the body. Here is a powerful pump that keeps the blood constantly circulating, endlessly traveling to even the most remote part of the body, and returning. The heart is a strong specialized muscle, one that endures a lot of activity and, when healthy, functions with ease and efficiency.

You will see, as you study the charts in Chapter 2, that the heart is located in the center of the chest, extending over to the left a bit. It is a two-way pumping station with four chambers. Two are receiving chambers for blood that enters the heart, and the other two pump blood away from the heart.

This organ is a very impressive pump that contracts forcefully. The right side of the heart is intense and contracts hard enough to send blood into the lungs.

However, it is the left side that is the most dominant, and its muscular contractions must be strong enough to send blood to every part of the body. Place your hand over your heart and you will feel your heartbeat; what you feel is the left side of the heart contracting. Keep this in mind when working the heart reflexes.

How Blood Is Recycled

Blood cells that have become deoxygenated return to the heart on the right side. These oxygen-poor cells are pumped through to the pulmonary artery at the top of the heart and carried into the lungs where they exchange carbon dioxide (waste gas) for new oxygen. The renewed oxygenated cells are then returned to the left side of the heart through the pulmonary veins. The left side of the heart then pumps the recycled, fully oxygenated blood through the aorta and into the rest of the body.

This oxygen-rich blood then travels through the circulatory system, carrying oxygen, hormones, nutrients, and even antibodies to cells in all parts of the body. This great circulatory river also transports waste products from the cells to distribution centers such as the lungs, liver, and kidneys. When it returns to the heart, this blood will be mostly depleted of oxygen again, and the process will repeat itself.

Coronary Circulation

The cardiac cycle is the time it takes between one heart contraction to the next. Each cycle is a natural action of the blood impulsively flowing through the heart chambers. Coronary circulation is important to the strength of the heart muscle; if the circulation system does not deliver the appropriate blood as needed, the result could be acute heart failure.

The Body's Natural Pacemaker

It is said that the heart produces an electrical current that controls its rhythmical contraction (heartbeat). The average adult has a rhythmic heart rate of about 72 beats per minute. This electrical wave also regulates the pace of blood flow as it is forced through the heart with enough push to reach all parts of the body.

Reflexology is based on balancing the body's systems so that they will ALL function in harmony. By stimulating the reflexes, we are sending vital energy into the zones to help the WHOLE BODY harmonize. This renewed stimulation will help unblock circulation pathways, activate nerve impulses, improve the blood supply, and normalize the balance of the entire body.

Use reflexology to keep this river of life constantly circulating within your veins, arteries, and through your heart. Your body will then be free of obstructions and your life full of joy and good health.

A Special Technique

Lift your leg up so that you can easily reach the left foot with the right hand. Keep in mind that you have already covered all of the chest area with reflexology, when you worked the lungs, thymus, solar plexus, bronchial, and stomach reflexes.

(If for some reason the reflex area of the chest was not stimulated earlier in the session, return to the chest and lung reflex areas to give them balanced stimulation. Work with a criss-cross technique across the foot from the instep to the outside edge, and back again. Criss-cross the heart reflex area on the left foot, as you did for the liver reflex on the right foot.)

Now it is time to concentrate on improving the rest of the circulatory system by sending energy to the arteries and veins, to break up any congestion that may be interfering with the vascular action of the heart.

With your right thumb, use heavy pressure, work along zones 3, 4, and 5, searching for the sore reflex that will tell you when you have reached the zone within which the trouble lies. This is frequently even more important than sending energy to the heart itself.

Good Circulation Is Critical

In review, the heart is an extraordinary pump that maintains blood circulation throughout the body. The blood travels on a round-trip cycle. Once it has been rejuvenated with oxygen, it is forced away from the heart through the main artery (the aorta). It travels through to smaller arteries and blood vessels, delivering oxygen to all cells and tissues throughout the body.

For purposes of illustration, let's say that these vessels are little "hoses" that carry the blood for miles, as they encircle the body. And let's compare the heart to other "pumps," such as a water pump or an air pump. If the hoses running from any one of these pumps become clogged, the narrowing hinders the flow, sometimes cutting it off completely.

It is the same with our circulatory system. If the veins or arteries become clogged, the blood cannot circulate through them to reach the heart. Good circulation is critical to the performance of the heart, as it is to all body functions, including our brain.

Notice in Photo 18, which illustrates the working of the heart and circulatory reflexes, that the thumb is pressed into the pad under the little toes, just as in reflexing the right foot for the liver reflex. Press and work this whole area, searching for tender spots. When you find any part that is tender, work it out, covering the area thoroughly. *If congestion in any degree is allowed to remain in the arteries and veins surrounding the heart, the result could be a heart attack.*

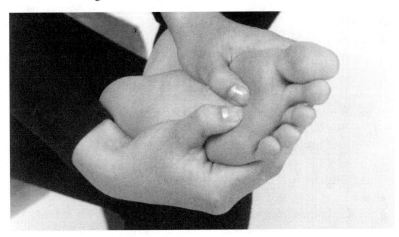

Photo 18. Double thumb action on the sole of foot is useful for working the large reflex area to the heart and vascular system. Also press-and-roll your fingers over top of foot with small circular movements for added stimulation to the chest area.

ANGINA PECTORIS

The distress from anginal pain is often a mild suffocating ache felt in the chest. Pain may also be felt in the neck, shoulder, and down the arm into the little finger. Often the upper part of the abdomen may feel the lack of sufficient oxygen, which will cause irritation and discomfort.

Anyone who has overexerted and started to feel dull pains in the left side of chest and down the left arm should stop and work the reflex areas shown, to stimulate the vascular system (because the heart is probably not getting enough blood). The body will benefit from both rest and working the reflexes.

Work the reflex areas that correspond to the coronary arteries, because this is where the heart gets its much needed blood. Also work the reflex areas that correspond to the zone in which the pain is felt. Use heavy pressure, and work both the top and sole of foot.

If the pain should increase or last longer than four, five or six minutes, it could be a heart attack, or even some other trouble. Always use common sense in a situation such as this; if you need a doctor, seek help wherever you can find it. Reflexology does not ever attempt to be considered as a substitute for needed medical care.

RELAXATION WITH REFLEXOLOGY

No matter what the nature of the trouble is, the heart can be aided with the "reflex push buttons." Reflexology is nature's natural tranquilizer; working the reflexes with slow, gentle movements will calm your entire system, and relax rigid muscles and veins.

How often I have helped someone with heart complaints by using reflexology while we waited for the doctor to arrive, or until I was satisfied the victim was out of danger and free from discomfort.

My reflexology instructor asked during class one day if any of her students, in the course of working on a person suffering from heart trouble, had noticed that person cry out when a sharp pain went from foot to heart, followed by the sensation of a stimulant. It was surprising to see over half the class signify that they had.

In my years of experience working on a person suffering from heart trouble, I have often seen this type of reaction, followed by the sensation of warmth, happiness and then complete relaxation.

Further investigation revealed that some cases showed the heart patient was never again troubled, even when the difficulties had been severe. If there is pain around the heart, or in the chest region, the entire area of reflexes, from the instep to the outside of foot, should be worked on. If the condition seems to be angina pectoris, characterized by pains going up the arm and shoulder, work clear to the base of the little toe and on top of it, as you would for the shoulder reflexes. Also work up to the root of the fourth and fifth toes to help unblock any obstructions that may be in the arteries or veins.

It should not take long to find the exact button which is crying for reflex stimulation to release the congestion.

SOME CAUSES OF DEATH FROM HEART TROUBLE

Probably too often death is declared to be from heart failure when actually it was the poor condition of other glands which caused the heart to give out from overwork.

People fill their bodies with unfit foods. They put an extra load on the heart by filling the lungs with nicotine. The list would be long if one were to jot down all the small items of daily living which tax the heart until it gives up. It is truly said that death overtakes one in "small bites."

This marvelous pumping station is located between the lungs and is enclosed in the cavity of the pericardium. It is embedded deep in the body. Often the reflex buttons will take more pressure than in other cases because of this. The heart covers quite an area in the upper portion of the chest cavity, slightly to the left. So there will be several reflex buttons, corresponding with the different parts of the heart and circulatory system around it.

If you are troubled with a heart condition, you will find it simpler to use the Reflex Massager, as it does the work of stimulating the reflexes with ease and puts no strain on you. Yes, it may be possible to reflex one's heartaches away!

CASES OF RECOVERIES FROM HEART TROUBLE

I can cite many case histories of wonderful results from this scientific technique of reflexology on heart patients. But this is one that I am going to give you as a warning. *Don't overdo! Never overdo!*

Mr. B. asked my help for a heart condition from which he had suffered for quite a while. With all his medicines, he was in and out of bed, and very weak from being inactive for so long. Remember that the heart is a muscle and when your outer muscles become flabby, so do the inner muscles, such as the heart. If your legs and arms were very soft from lying around for several months, you wouldn't try to go out and play several games of tennis, ball, or golf, just because you felt good one day, would you? If you did, you would probably have muscle spasms in your arms and legs all night.

Now the heart is a muscle, too, a big muscle. Twenty-four quarts of blood pass through the circulatory system in three minutes. In a male, the heart weighs from 10 to 12 ounces in proportion to the size of the body. If you overtax it with unusual exercise before giving it a chance to build up strength after a long rest, it could very easily have a muscle spasm, too—heart attack! This often happens to people who have been retired or inactive for a number of months, then go on a trip which requires a lot of activity.

Mr. B. took about three treatments from me in a period of seven days. He felt so well that he decided he would go to work. He was sure he was well, which he certainly could have been, but his heart was still very soft from months of inactivity. I told him repeatedly, "Wait a while, give yourself time to get strong, don't rush it. Give your heart a chance." That same week he went to the factory to ask for his old job back. He drove the car over 100 miles. He felt like a new man, he said. He walked all over the big factory, up many flights of stairs and down again.

His old boss was glad to have him back and was showing him around. On the way back to the car he had to walk up a long hill, and this is when his heart began to protest. After that he was back to his old up-and-down routine. He never came back to me. He lost faith in this great work that might have made him a healthy man the rest of his life. If he had only listened to my warning, or even used common sense!

Don't you be a Mr. B., no matter how well you get to feeling after working your reflexes. Take a little time, give your body a chance to build up strength and muscle, and you will be able to stay "regenerated" all of your life.

Case History of Heart and Stress Conditions Eased

Mr. H. came to me with several complaints, the most pressing of which was a heart condition caused by rheumatic fever which he had suffered when he was a child. In addition he had a nervous stomach. He had spent much of his time in hospitals and had been bedfast for months at a time. He was married, with several children to support, and this affliction made life very hard on him and his family. Luckily he owned his own business, but it suffered setbacks when he had attacks and would have to remain in bed for several weeks at a time. This caused him to go into a mental depression which, in addition to his heart condition, caused a vicious circle of disharmony in the body.

His nerves were in terrible condition and he was plainly under strong mental stress. In fact, he had become so bad that he would have crying spells for no reason. He could not relax enough to fall asleep at night, which added to his condition because we all know that the body heals while we sleep. He had no appetite, showing a depression of digestive activities. He suffered from constipation. In plain words, he was a physical wreck and the only future he had to look forward to was to get worse and to finally end up in an early grave.

Mr. H. was only in his early 30's at the time he came to me for reflex sessions to see if I could bring him some relief for his stomach, since eating had become a serious problem.

You have probably known people like this who seem to go from bad to worse, at last hopelessly giving up life. Mr. H. proceeded to tell me of all his ailments and complaints as I started to reflex his very tender feet. He wouldn't have had to tell me his problems because they were all there reflecting in the bottoms of his feet. I felt that they were screaming for help as I worked each reflex very gently. With a warm feeling of pleasure, I watched this poor, distressed man quiet down as I worked on the reflexes, especially those to the endocrine glands. Remember, I had to be very careful not to overwork any particular reflex area the first time due to his bad condition, so I spent a few minutes just rubbing the whole foot with my open hand while I watched him drop off to sleep for a few minutes.

It was a pleasure to watch Mr. H. regaining his health, as the stimulation of working the reflexes started his congested glands and organs back to normal functioning. I renewed the circulation in his whole body by working all of the reflexes in both feet. Thus not just one of his many symptoms began to show improvement, but we were rewarded by his overall return to health.

When he first came to me he had been despondent and without hope. Yet after the first session his wife noticed his renewed sense of well being. Almost at once his disposition improved and she told me later that instead of crying, he was cheerful and better natured than she had seen him since their early marriage. And she said he would fall asleep as soon as his head hit the pillow, something that he had not been able to do for years.

All of this added up to an increase of vitality in the whole mechanism of his body. His stomach improved rapidly and he was able to eat again without discomfort as soon as the disturbances of the digestive tract had been helped back to a normal functioning when stimulated by the reflexes.

As his glands began to respond to the stimulation, Mr. H.'s whole body took on new life. He found that he was no longer constipated and could give up taking harsh laxatives. And as each organ and gland relaxed, it freed his mind from mental and nervous tension. As the system recuperated and became stronger, so did his heart.

Doctors had always warned him that he could not do the things other men did. He must remain a semi-invalid all of his life if he wanted to live at all. What a joy it was when his heart returned to normal, enough to allow him to do anything that he wanted to do without any trouble. His blood pressure returned to normal; his eyes sparkled with health and joy for the first time since he was a small boy.

Today, after more than ten years, he is a strong and well man, running a large, successful business and enjoying sports in his spare time.

What did I do to make a new man of Mr. H.? Well, the first thing that I worked on was the reflex to the pituitary/hypothalamus gland which, if you remember your chart, is in the center of the big toe. These are the main glands of the whole body—the "king" glands.

Then I dropped on down to the reflex of the thyroid which is just below the big toe; next I reflexed the thymus for a few seconds; then on down the foot to the adrenal reflexes; and on down to the pancreas; from there to the gonads or sex glands under the ankles; then my fingers searched out the reflexes to the spleen, which is the storehouse of energy and the red blood builder. I went from one foot to the other, making sure I only pressed on each reflex two or three times at the most.

I stimulated the endocrine glands first. Then I carefully worked on the rest of the reflexes, such as heart, liver, kidneys, and the eyes and ear area and the sinus reflexes, because he was also afflicted with a bad case of sinus trouble. The whole body was out of harmony, out of tune, and we merely helped nature put it back in tune by working the reflexes and giving her a chance to bring new life to all of the congested glands and dying cells in the body. Thus health was quickly and simply restored through the wonder of reflexology.

LEARN TO RECOGNIZE THE SIGNS OF HEART TROUBLES

Many different things can contribute to an ill heart. It would help you to learn how to recognize symptoms that signal cardiovascular problems. As you become acquainted with them you will be better prepared for an emergency should one occur. Read all you can and get a clear visual picture of what you would do in case of an emergency. Learning how the heart functions, and signs of various symptoms, could save the life of someone you care about. Here is a list of conditions to help you understand the heart's complexity.

- *Circulatory Problems* cause many disorders, including high blood pressure and hypertension. Hardening of the arteries results from lack of good circulation, as do fatty deposits along the arterial walls. And you remember that slow circulation is one cause of strokes or anginal attacks. Take an active part in protecting your family's health: use reflexology and get family members involved in activities that keep blood circulation moving.
- *Arteriosclerosis* is hardening of the arteries, and obstructs the flow of blood, resulting in a heart attack. (Symptoms: deep intense pain in chest, possible shortness of breath, difficulty in swallowing, sweating, and dizziness. Other signs include nausea or vomiting, ringing in the ears, inability to talk, a feeling of fear, possibly even fainting.)
- *Angina Pectoris* occurs when the heart is getting insufficient amounts of oxygen, usually after exertion of some sort. (Symptoms: profound pains felt in chest, and sometimes in the jaw, neck, shoulder, and left arm down to the little finger.)
- *Arrhythmias* occur when the heartbeat has a disturbance in its natural rhythm, due to an electrical (natural pacemaker) disruption. (Symptoms: heart beats out of sequence, possible feeling that the heart is fluttering or is skipping a beat.)
- *Hypertension* is high blood pressure and, if untreated, could result in a stroke or cause heart problems.

- *Stroke* is a vascular condition which affects the blood supply to the brain. The artery to the brain may get clogged, which cuts off oxygen to a section of the brain. (Symptoms: numbness in face, arm or loss of vision on one side of body, possible headache, dizziness or inability to stand up, difficulty in understanding what another person is saying, or loss of speech.)
- *Artery Blood Clot* occurs when blood congeals in the artery and cuts off circulation to the heart, causing damage to the heart.
- *Cardiac Arrest* is when the heart stops beating. The blood supply therefore does not go to the brain and the result is dizziness and subsequent loss of consciousness.
- *Congestive Heart Failure* occurs when a heart that is already damaged becomes exhausted. Often fluid gets in the lungs and it's hard to breathe. (Symptoms: check for swollen ankles and feet, a general feeling of fatigue, abnormal breathing, possible excessive gas and nausea.)

PREVENTION IS THE KEY TO A STRONG AND HEALTHY CARDIOVASCULAR SYSTEM

Since cardiovascular disease is a leading health problem universally, let's do whatever we can to improve oxygen supply to the heart and keep our circulation moving. There are many natural ways, such as the following ten suggestions, to help prevent heart and vascular problems.

Ten Effective Steps to Help Maintain a Healthy Heart

1. Reflexology is one effective way to improve internal functioning by helping the body keep its circulatory system invigorated. The heart must be kept busy, circulating blood to all areas of the body and brain. If it slows down, the lifelines of circulation also slow down and deterioration can set in. Focus on the reflex areas of the circulation system to strengthen an ailing heart.
2. Exercise is important, so move your body whenever you can. Stretch your arms above your chest, out to your sides, and in big

circles. Make the circles out to the sides of your body; first move them clockwise, then counter-clockwise, then follow by placing them both in front of you and draw a big number 8 in the air. The next day, do two of each exercise and add to the regimen some of your own inventive movements, such as using both hands to draw big letters in the air (spell out your name, your animals' names or draw the alphabet). Remember, do not over-do at first. Gradually work up to additional movements; when you feel tired, sit down and rest.

3. Walking is nature's natural stimulator. Walking briskly and swinging your arms at your sides for about twenty minutes, five or six times a week is good for cardiac and arterial health. If the weather is terrible outside, you can walk to the beat of music, or count your steps as you walk around the house, moving your arms and legs to improve your circulation. Better circulation means a stronger heart muscle.

4. Use the Deluxe-Foot-Roller to increase your circulation and get your blood moving. When using this helpful tool, you are moving your legs and feet which encourages the blood to circulate throughout your whole body.

5. Walk around the house without your shoes on to stimulate the reflexes in your feet naturally. If you get a feeling like pins and needles, you can be sure that the reflexes are telling you that there is impaired blood circulation somewhere in your body.

6. There are various causes of blood pressure troubles. You can relieve stress and tension with reflexology and visualization; here's one suggestion. Make yourself comfortable; gently work over the reflexes in your feet and let your mind drift off. Your whole body will feel the healing forces of nature being stimulated through the reflexes. Picture yourself in a pleasant, peaceful place and imagine enjoyable sounds and smells. Breathe rhythmically from your diaphragm as you relax totally. (If you are at work, take a break from any challenging situations, close your eyes, use visualization and deep breathing exercise while you softly work the reflexes in your hands.) As your mind becomes calm and relaxed, feel the magical vibrations of reflexology releasing all tensions from your body, bringing down any rise in blood pressure.

7. Avoid gaining weight. Overweight is a big risk factor both for heart attacks and for high blood pressure. Also avoid salt and products that contain sodium.

8. If you have a serious heart problem and are on medications, it is important to know what prescriptions you may need in case of emergency. Share this information with someone nearby; also write it down. Have telephone numbers of friends, family members, or emergency close by.

9. Watch your diet by eliminating caffeine, fried, and processed foods. Avoid foods high in fats (especially animal fats) and cholesterol. If you are still smoking, try very hard to stop, as nicotine does constrict circulation. Eat foods that are good for your heart, such as fish, whole grains, raw foods, fresh greens, onions, and garlic. Studies have found that marine lipids (fish oils) and omega 3, both fatty acids, are healthy for the heart. Vitamins such as lecithin and Vitamin E (Vitamin E helps digest lecithin), B complex, potassium, magnesium, Ester C and antioxidants such as CoQ 10 are beneficial in the diet. These helpful preventatives can be found wherever vitamins are sold.

10. Daily prevention should include some deep breathing exercises to give your body the oxygen it needs. Watch a funny movie or read the comics whenever you can, and laugh at every amusing moment; this will enrich your lungs with renewed oxygen. Merriment is very relaxing, which will help keep the blood pressure down. Giving your respiratory, as well as your circulatory system, some exercise will help regenerate your healthy heart.

CHAPTER 16

Reflexing the Appendix and Ileocecal Valve

Location of ILEOCECAL Valve and APPENDIX within right side of body.

APPENDIX and ILEOCECAL Valve reflex area in right foot.

The appendix is one of the best-known organs, although it is a tube no more than 3 to 6 inches long lying below the waist near the juncture of the small and large intestines and on the right side of the body.

PROPER REFLEX TECHNIQUES

To work this reflex, let's take a look at Photo 19 for position of reflexes to the appendix and ileocecal valve. Notice how the thumb is pressed in about three-quarters of the way down the foot from the toes, and quite close to the outer edge of the foot. To locate the reflex to this wormlike organ, you will have to do a little exploring. If there is no congestion in the appendix or inflammation in the ileocecal valve, then you will not be able to find it. But don't worry because they are so centrally located that their reflexes will get enough stimulation to keep them in good, healthy condition.

To work the appendix reflex, which you know will be on the right foot as the appendix is on the right side of the body, lift the right foot into position as shown in Photo 19. Now press in the area shown in the picture with a rolling motion, until you hit the button under the skin that will give you the pain signal that there is trouble here.

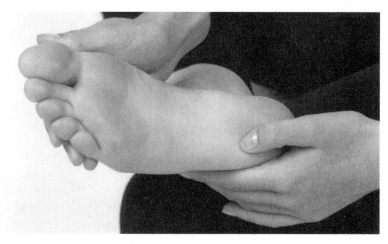

Photo 19. Position for reaching the reflexes to the appendix and ileocecal valve.

You will probably have to move your thumb, or reflex tool, around a bit on this particular reflex before you find it.

It seems to be in a little different area on different people, but not over a quarter of an inch one way or the other. When you do find it, work the tender reflex for a few seconds; then let it rest while you work some other area. Then come back to it and reflex a few more seconds. Do this each time you work your reflexes until all tenderness has vanished.

REPORTED RECOVERIES FROM APPENDICITIS

Many marvelous recoveries from appendicitis have been experienced because of working the reflexes for this organ. In case of an acute attack, the attention of a physician would be needed, of course. However, you may cautiously work the appendix reflex until medical care is given, as it will relax the inflamed area involved.

A friend of mine did not believe in this reflex system of healing for herself, although she sent many of her friends to me for treatments. One day I went to visit her and found her lying on her bed in much pain. "I've got appendicitis," she moaned. "Call the doctor!" I said, "I will not call the doctor until you let me see your feet. I don't believe you have appendicitis at all." I went over and picked up her right foot, pressed on the reflex to the appendix, and found there was no tenderness. Then I moved up to the reflex of the stomach and solar plexus and found this area somewhat tender. I worked it for just a few seconds; she expelled some gas, and the pain was completely gone. She couldn't believe that the pain had disappeared so suddenly.

From then on, when I went to see her she would kick off her shoes so I could give her feet some stimulation.

THE IMPORTANT ILEOCECAL VALVE

Tenderness in this particular region of the foot, however, can sometimes indicate trouble other than in the appendix. The ileocecal valve forms the opening from the small intestine into the colon. This opening is toward the large intestine and guards against reflex from the large into the small bowel. This is an important area, especially if you are inclined to suffer from an allergy.

A CASE OF FOOD ALLERGY HEALED

Mr. C. had been a seaman all his life and enjoyed his work, but through the years he had developed an allergy to various foods served at sea. At first he did not pay much attention to the distress, but as time passed he became increasingly worse until it seemed that everything he ate made him break out with hives or gave him indigestion. Finally he had to give up his life on the seas—he had reached the point where he was afraid to eat anything. Doctors had given him tests, and he had been taking shots and pills until he said he had become allergic even to them. He had tried everything else, he told me, and wanted to see if reflexology was the answer.

When I took his feet in my hands, I found all of the reflexes extremely tender. After carefully working the endocrine reflexes for a few seconds, I moved my fingers to the spot under the second toe (from the big toe). This was so tender that he could barely stand to have me touch it, but using my "feather touch" I worked on all the toes, one by one, rolling and twisting them gently between my fingers.

Then I concentrated on the *ileocecal valve* reflex. This is located in the same position as the appendix reflex, and he moaned out loud with pain as my fingers barely pressed the spot. Notice in Chart B how this reflex is situated slightly toward the outer edge from the center of the foot.

When Mr. C. got home, he called me to tell me that he already felt much better, and that he was confident he would recover his health.

When he came back in two days, he looked so much better that I was amazed at the change. He had lost his gray color, and his face was no longer drawn and haggard. He said he had slept soundly for the past two nights, and though he was still wary about food, his meals had caused him little distress.

It was surprising to see how few reflex sessions it took to put Mr. C. back on the road to living a healthy, normal life once more. He insists that reflexology saved his very life. Now, several years later, he is completely free of all food allergies, eats whatever he wants to, and enjoys perfect health, all thanks to nature's own simple way of restoring the organs and glands to normalcy.

CASE HISTORY OF A SINUS CONDITION HEALED

Mr. M. came to me with a bad case of sinus. His head had become so stuffed up that he was unable to go to work for days at a time. A businessman who had to face the public, he was embarrassed when he could not close his mouth, but had to keep it open in order to breathe.

Of course, he had all of the other symptoms that go with sinuses, such as headaches, poor hearing at times, nervousness and irritability, upset stomach, etc. Naturally the reflexes indicated all of this the first time I gave him reflexology.

After I had gone over both of his feet and worked each and every tender reflex, I concentrated on the ileocecal valve reflex located in the same area as that to the appendix, on the right foot, a little up toward the toes from the center of the foot and just a little toward the outside of the foot.

If you are bothered with sinus of any kind, you will have no trouble in locating this reflex, as it will shock you with pain when it is pressed firmly with the thumb or a like self-help tool. Press in deeply enough to reach the button under the skin.

Next I worked all of the reflexes under the toes, which were extremely sore, especially the one just at the bottom of the second toe. This reflex seems to be the main one that will loosen the congestion of sinus in the head, and it doesn't seem to matter how long this particular reflex is worked if you are careful not to bruise the capillaries (tiny blood vessels) in the skin.

I noticed Mr. M. seemed to be getting relief on the left side of his head as I worked the reflexes in the left foot. Suddenly he could breathe through his nostril on the left side. "Boy, what a relief," he exclaimed.

Then I went to work on the right foot and reflexed under the toes again as I had done on the left foot. After some time of reflexing, the right side of his head opened up so that he was able to also breathe through the right nostril. He was so elated and surprised at the results, he said, "I didn't really believe this would help when I came in here. I almost canceled the appointment, it seemed so ridiculous."

I laughingly told him that I had heard those same words many times. But the sad thing was some people actually did back out at the last minute from lack of faith in the method of reflexology; that has always made me feel bad for that person who had come so close to such a simple and natural way back to health and then missed it.

After I had helped Mr. M. breathe normally again, I asked him about his back. I had noticed that it was extremely tender in one area, as I had been covering his reflexes in the general workout.

He told me that he had a slipped disc, according to the doctors, and that it was getting worse fast. The doctors had told him that nothing but an operation could help him, and that it was a very serious and dangerous operation. He said that he knew he was going to have to give up and have it done soon, but dreaded it. "Too bad these treatments aren't magic enough to fix my back, too," he said jokingly.

"What makes you think they can't?" I asked him. "You didn't believe that they could help your sinuses an hour ago, and look at you now! Why couldn't they do as much for your back or any other part of your body for that matter?"

He looked at me in real surprise. "You mean they really could?" he asked in amazement. "Don't you think that they could?" I asked him seriously. "Yes, I do believe they can if you say so; after relieving my sinuses with reflex therapy, I would believe that they could do anything. I will come back every day for additional reflex help," he said. I had to explain to him that one treatment every other day was all that he should take, for the first week anyway.

Mr. M. came faithfully every other day during the first week, then one day a week. Sometimes his wife would call me early in the morning to ask if I would give Mr. M. a treatment for his sinus condition so he could go to work that day, when he would have an attack between sessions. His allergies did not vanish in a week. His body had taken a long time to get into that state, and it took a little while to put it back into a condition that was once more in tune with the universe.

Remember this truth if your health does not become perfect as soon as you want it to. It must have been neglected for a long time, so be patient and persevere. So don't forget to use nature's reflexes as the way to keep the circulation flowing freely, to loosen and banish all congestion from the body.

When Mr. M. came over for special workouts on his sinus reflexes, I concentrated on the toes. Sometimes I would work the reflex at the base of the second and third toes for over an hour before we could break the congestion loose, but when we finally succeeded he was able to go to work free from any signs of congestion in his head, often remaining so for some time.

As we kept up the reflex sessions, he noticed a great improvement in his back also. Within a year he was able to take long hikes up and down mountains, carrying large, bulky backpacks. He was able to paint his home, climbing ladders and carrying paint, etc. And in two years he roofed his house, carrying heavy bundles of roofing up high ladders, with no recurrences of the back trouble he had complained of before he had reflexology.

Don't underestimate the power of reflexology no matter what your complaint. It cannot hurt to try, and your reward will most likely be a satisfactory recovery.

CHAPTER 17

How to Reflex the Small and Large Intestines

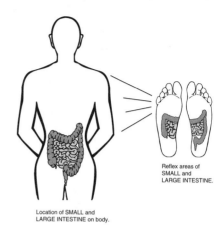

Location of SMALL and LARGE INTESTINE on body.

Reflex areas of SMALL and LARGE INTESTINE.

This chapter discusses the small and large intestines. First, let's study the small intestine. Notice in Chart A at the beginning of this book how it seems to fill the lower abdomen. This intestine is the longest of the gastrointestinal tract, a channel so coiled and twisted upon itself that it winds and bends for more than 20 feet.

The food that you have swallowed and taken into the stomach passes on into this twenty feet of intestine. Pushed slowly through by the muscle walls, it is broken up by enzymes until well digested. Useful food particles are then absorbed by the bloodstream, and the waste passes down to the large intestine.

If you feel there is congestion in the small intestine, work this whole area thoroughly. You will be amazed how quickly reflexology will bring relief from gastric pain, disturbances, and flatulence.

SPECIAL REFLEX TECHNIQUES FOR THE SMALL INTESTINE

Note that the reflexes to the small intestine are located in the heel, and because they cover such a large area it is wise to reflex the whole pad of the heel. You will also note in Chart A how the colon makes almost a complete circle around the small intestine. Keep this in mind when working the reflexes to the small intestine, which are found from the waistline down to the heel, and all the way across from the inside almost to the outside of the foot.

Let's start by taking one foot up into position and, with a deep rolling motion, work from just below the waistline down to the heel. Work back and forth across the foot until you get down to the bottom of the heel. Since the heel area has a heavier layer of skin and is usually quite thick, use the knuckle of a finger, or a reflex tool, to press in deeply enough to do some good, especially if you feel there is congestion.

When using the Reflex Probe, use the blunt side to cover the whole area more completely. If you find pinpoints of tenderness, continue to work the buttons under the skin with the blunt tip; however, if you find that the blunt tip is not reaching the reflexes, then turn the probe over and use the sharper end. The Reflex Roller can be a big help in your routine, because it will be easy to roll over the whole heel area.

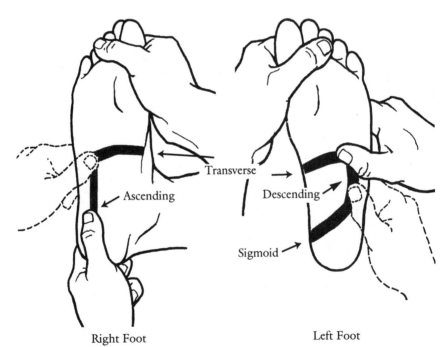

Right Foot   Left Foot

Illustration 16a. Follow the course of the colon: Work the ascending and transverse colon reflex area on your right foot.

Illustration 16b. Work the transverse, descending and sigmoid colon reflex area on your left foot.

THE LARGE INTESTINE

Now we come to the large intestine, more commonly known as the colon, in tracing the intestinal system. The small intestine deposits the waste of our food into the large intestine or colon, where it is forced through to the rectum, and by a series of final contractions is forced from the body as wastes.

The colon is about twice the diameter of the small intestine; however, it is only about five or six feet long. The site of the first part of the colon is best known because the appendix opens into it close to the junction with the small intestine and the ileocecal valve. We have already seen on Chart A how the wormlike appendix is attached and how the colon stretches upward from the right lower corner of the abdomen. From there it curves just below the liver to course across the upper abdomen as the transverse colon, descending on the left side to bend into the coils of what is called the sigmoid flexure, and from there joins the rectum.

How the Colon Works

Bacteria are numerous in the colon. Their presence is important to the body because of their ability to build up such essential substances as vitamin K, needed for blood coagulation, and several components of vitamin B. At times the continuous taking of antibacterial drugs, which sterilize the intestine, has resulted in vitamin K deficiency.

The colon is the final canal for food passage. What remains of the food solution spends 10 to 12 hours in the large intestine, losing large quantities of water. As a final step, the solution is attacked by a colony of bacteria to decay the remains of what started out as a meal.

This is the garbage pail of the body, and is truly the seat of many illnesses. It should be emptied for good health at least once or twice a day as animals do.

Colon Reflex Techniques

Let us start reflexing the colon by lifting the right foot up into position, since the colon has its beginning at the end of the small intestine low down on the right side of the abdomen. With the thumb of the left hand, press near the outside of the foot on the pad of the heel and work up toward the waistline of the foot with a pressing-rolling motion.

I suggest that you use the thumb of the left hand for this position, as it seems to give you more power than you would have with the right thumb. You will soon learn which position is the most convenient for you—use it. Simplify most of your work done on thick skin using a self-help reflex tool.

Work your way up to the waistline of the foot, still using your pressing-rolling motion; go across the foot toward the center and work to the reflexes of the spine. Work this area several times, hunting for buttons that will give you pain signals telling you if something is wrong. When you do find these tender spots, reflex them a few seconds each. Keep in mind that pain suggests congestion; working that particular reflex will release a supply of life-giving blood, hastening the healing process and relieving the congested tissues.

Now we have the remainder of the colon on the left side of the body, as you will see in the illustration on page 132. Lift the left leg up into position. Use the left thumb to start reflexing the buttons on this foot. It will be best to start at the waistline of the foot on the inside next to the reflexes of the spine and work toward the outer edge of the foot, as we follow the colon in its natural travel across the foot toward the descending colon.

When you come to the outside of the foot, change hands; it will be easier to use your right thumb to reflex the descending colon. Continue the same rolling-pressing motion (or use the press-and-pull-down technique you learned from page 47, Chapter 5).

Work down the outside of the left foot, and back across the pad of the heel to the inside of the foot, following the course of the descending and sigmoid colon in the body. You will change hands a few times here. Use the one that is more natural to you for reaching this lengthy reflex area.

You may find some spots along here that will make you wince with pain at the slightest pressure. Reflex them gently at first, increasing the pressure as the pain subsides. You cannot be sure whether it is the colon or perhaps some other organ that is sending out the pain messages as you reflex over certain areas, especially along the transverse section. Don't let this concern you; just keep in mind that where congestion exists, disease will result. Work it out.

As a world-famous surgeon, the late Sir W.A. Lane, said: "There is but one disease, insufficient drainage—inadequate elimination of poisonous waste material. Unless it is thrown off, poisonous waste remains in the system and begins slowly to undermine the health of our organism, finally destroying it." Is this happening to you? If so, now you know what to do about it.

Varicose Veins

Varicose veins are also helped through working the colon and the liver reflexes. I have brought lasting relief to sufferers of varicose veins by starting the proper circulation with reflexology, thus causing the congestion to disappear. This is true also with cramps or pains of any kind in the legs.

Dear Mrs. Carter,

Health and vitality can be restored through reflexology. For myself, it is giving me a feeling of self-worth. I absolutely love to be able to help people in this way. Reflexology is totally awesome (how it relates to the body, etc.), but at the same time actually simple in that it is drug-free and just helping to aid the body do its natural thing! We are wonderfully made.

The colon is the seat of many illnesses; reflexology is beneficial to unblocking the congestion. Also varicose veins can be helped through working the reflexes of the colon and liver. I am SO HAPPY to be able to learn this technique. If more people were aware of reflexology and tried it, I'm sure a lot of surgery could be avoided! I can't tell you how grateful I am. Thank you, Mildred Carter, I would love to meet you in person! Maybe someday I will.

—Ms. P.F., Alabama

CHAPTER 18

Reflex to the Bladder

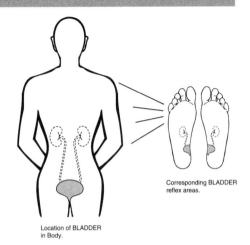

Corresponding BLADDER
reflex areas.

Location of BLADDER
in Body.

The bladder is a hollow muscular sac into which the ureters empty.
The ureters are two hollow, thin-walled tubes about the caliber of a
pencil which connect the kidneys to the bladder, one tube coming
from each kidney. Urine cannot run down the ureter by gravity, since
passage through it must continue even when we are lying down.
Urine is moved along by peristalsis, waves of contracting circular muscle similar to those that expel material from the bronchi or the intestine.

The bladder, whose function it is to store urine for periodic
release, changes position and shape according to the amount of filling. When it is empty, the bladder is flat or concave on top and
inclines forward. When it is full, it becomes rounded and projects
upward. It is composed of a smooth muscle coat like that of the intestine, but of greater thickness. The urethra is the tubelike passage
which conducts the urine from the bladder and expels it to the exte-
rior.

TECHNIQUES FOR BLADDER REFLEX

Study Chart A and notice how the bladder lies in the lower lumbar
region. Its reflexes will be in the same place as those to the end of the

136

spine, only not so deep. Notice in Photo 20 the position of the thumb, and how it is pressed into the soft, hollow part on the inside of the foot, almost next to the pad of the heel. You will be able to feel a soft, spongy area about as large as a quarter. The thumb is positioned to stimulate the bladder reflex. With a rolling-pressing motion, work the thumb on up the ureter tube to the kidney reflex. Repeat this a few times also.

Lift either foot up into position. The reflex to the bladder will be on both feet in the same location, since the bladder is located in the center of the body. Now the foot is ready to be reflexed. You will notice in the picture that we again use the hand on the same side as the foot we are reflexing—right foot, right hand, left foot, left hand. The thumb will press into the bladder reflex almost naturally. Work with a gentle, circular motion, concentrating on any part that is tender.

If you are having trouble with the bladder and do not seem to find a tender spot in this area, keep pressing a little deeper until you do touch the reflex button, which will give you a pain signal that you are on the right spot. This reflex is so near the location of the rectum, prostate, and lower spine reflexes that you will not be able to tell the difference except for the depth of the reflex work. For these reflexes you will probably have to use the Reflex Probe or like tool in order to press hard enough to reach these particular buttons. It's just like reaching through the front of your pelvis to reach the end of the spine. The reflex to your rectum will be toward the back of the heel just a bit.

BLADDER DISORDERS HELPED

Work the whole spongy area for the bladder reflex on the surface. Cystitis (inflammation of the bladder) will work out very quickly and usually you will notice a great improvement after the first reflex workout. All sensation of burning and itching usually disappears completely after the second or third workout. Any sensation of irritation in the bladder area will be benefited by working these reflexes. Remember, if at any time in any area there is bleeding, and it persists after the third workout or after a week of treatments, consult your physician to make sure there is no malignancy present.

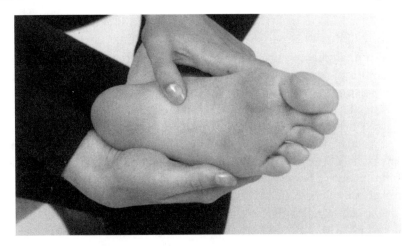

Photo 20. Support your foot with one hand. Use thumb of opposite hand to work the soft spongy area just above the heel on the inside of your foot. Thumb-walk between the kidney and bladder reflexes.

I have had so many wonderful results from working the reflexes to the bladder, by relaxing tension and breaking up congestion, allowing normal circulation to flow through the cells as nature intended. You can have the same results by following the directions carefully.

Case History of Bladder Trouble Healed

A woman had a chronic weakness in her bladder so troublesome that she would often have to go to bed. She took various medicines which gave only temporary relief.

She decided to try reflexology and called me to see if I would schedule her a course of reflex sessions. She was not expecting any real help, I knew by her voice on the phone, but she was coming to me as a last try for relief. This was nothing new to me as a lot of people only try reflexology after everything else fails.

When I started to work on her feet, I found that the reflex to the pituitary was so tender that I could hardly touch her big toe. I had to hold it in the palm of my hand for a few minutes before I could even work it. I had a hard time talking her into letting me continue with the session when she found out it was going to hurt.

If you find that some of the reflexes are so tender that you cannot touch them even with a "feather touch," then try holding the palm of your hand over the area for a few minutes; some of the soreness will abate enough so that you can work it lightly at first.

I worked the big toe lightly, then moved on down to the thyroid reflex under the bone of the big toe. This also was very tender, and so were the adrenal reflexes in the center of her feet. In fact, all of the endocrine glands were terribly congested according to the messages the reflexes sent out. No wonder her bladder was always infected. It was a wonder she didn't have many other symptoms to warn her that her body was completely out of harmony. She admitted that she had felt ill for quite some time but had laid the blame on the bladder trouble. Thus the bladder is all that she had ever doctored, although her trouble was much deeper than chronic bladder infection. It was not possible for the bladder to heal until she got to the cause of the trouble.

I explained to her what each reflex was and the gland to which it corresponded, as well as how it stimulated that certain gland with new circulation, bringing it back to life. She became very interested and could even feel little shock vibrations in some of the places in her body as I worked on the reflexes to them. I didn't reflex any one place on her feet more than a few seconds, except the area of the bladder, because she was too full of congestion in all of the glands to take a chance of loosening too much poison into her system at once. I worked the bladder reflex on each foot a few minutes until some of the tenderness was worked out.

She was so amazed at the improvement she felt upon getting out of the chair that she couldn't believe it was true.

It took about five sessions in all, and she never had another occurrence of bladder infection. She regained her original pep and vigor and looked and felt ten years younger within a month after starting the reflexology sessions.

I advised her to continue reflexing her own feet to keep her systems balanced and her bladder free from being overworked.

CHAPTER 19

Reflexes to Sex Glands and Organs

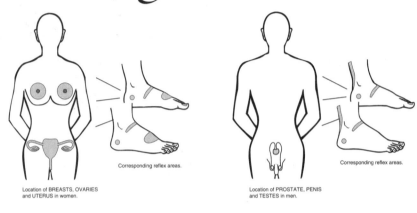

Corresponding reflex areas.

Location of BREASTS, OVARIES and UTERUS in women.

Corresponding reflex areas.

Location of PROSTATE, PENIS and TESTES in men.

The reflexes of the gonads, or sex glands, in both male and female are very important. The testes of men and the ovaries of women are associated almost exclusively with their reproductive functions. While reproduction is unquestionably the most important function of the gonads, the hormones which they produce have far-reaching effects on the body generally, and even upon mental activity.

Certain distinct cells of the ovaries and testes devote themselves to the production of steroid hormones, while others evolve into spermatozoa and ova. Both functions are closely related to and controlled by the pituitary gland.

Study Chart E on endocrine glands and Chart C in the beginning of the book and you will see the position of the sex organs, as well as that of the reflexes. Nature has seen fit to move the reflexes to these most important glands up above the soles of the feet, maybe to protect them from overstimulation when people walked on their bare feet, as they were intended to do in the beginning of time.

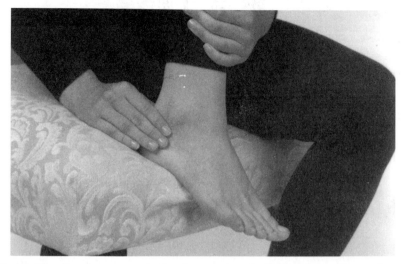

Photo 21. Gently rotate two fingers, or thumb, below the ankle on the outside of the foot for reflexes to the ovaries and fallopian tubes in women, (or) testes in men.

Now let us look at Photos 21 and 22. In these areas under the ankles you will find the reflexes to the ovaries, uterus, and fallopian tubes in the female; and the testicles, penis, and prostate glands in the male. Many reflexes are centered around the ankles, understandable since there are a lot of glands and organs of the reproductive system close together in the body.

SPECIAL REFLEX TECHNIQUES

On the *outside* of each foot, just under the ankle bone, is the reflex to the ovaries and fallopian tubes in the female, and the testicles in the male. As usual, the right foot corresponds to the right side of the body, and the left foot to the left side.

By looking at Chart C we see that the female uterus and the male prostate and penis reflexes are found under the ankle on the *inside* of the foot.

There will probably be some extremely tender spots in several places of this area, on both male and female, since this will cover the reflexes to all of the organs, glands, muscles, and veins in the lower section of the body that are centrally located.

When there is inflammation in any part of the lower abdomen, you may feel like you have one big ache, from the navel down to the lowest region. No matter what is congested, a surge of stimulation can be started by working the reflexes that are tender, thus equalizing the circulation and restoring health.

Reflexing the Ovaries or Testes

In Photo 21, notice how the foot is pulled back and the index and middle fingers are pressed together just below the ankle and above the heel bone. You can also work this area using your thumb, moving it in a slow circular motion. Or you may lift the leg up on your lap as we have been doing, if it is more comfortable for you. In this position, you will use the fingers of the opposite hand to press under the ankle. Use a very gentle rolling motion in this whole area under the ankle, concentrating on extremely tender spots. This area will generally be quite tender to most people.

Reflexology has brought relief to many for several different complaints. These include puberty difficulties, irregular or painful menstruation problems, swollen ankles, severe mood swings, and premenstrual syndrome. It will not prevent menopause from occurring, as this is a normal cycle of life. However, the challenges often accompanied

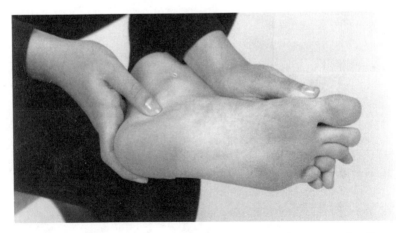

Photo 22. Use your thumb, or two fingers, to gently press-and-roll on the inside of foot under ankle bone, and down toward the back of heel. This is the position for working the reflexes to the uterus in women (or) the penis and prostate gland in men.

by the reduction of hormone production, such as hot flashes and depression, have been helped immensely.

Men have been freed from vague aches and pains, insomnia, sexual performance difficulties, and prostate troubles. I work on all of the reflexes, but very lightly and only twenty seconds on the area under the ankles, on the inside and the outside of the feet.

I work over the top of the foot also, from one ankle to the other, because this is an assistant reflex to the groin area, as well as the best reflex area to circulate the lymphatic system. It is also beneficial with any troubles of the sex glands to work all of the endocrine glands, the lower back, and the lower abdomen reflexes on both feet.

When you have the opportunity to use reflexology for the health of these glands, you will notice how quickly stress and fatigue in these areas vanish.

Reflexing the Uterus or Penis and Prostate Gland

Take the left foot up into position for reflexing. See Photo 22. Notice how the thumb of the right hand presses between the ankle and the heel on the inside of the left foot.

Press firmly with a rolling circular motion of the thumb, moving back and forth, being sure to cover the entire area under the ankle. Give special attention to the very tender places, keeping in mind that some of these reflexes are tiny, pinpoint spots and the area must be covered thoroughly. Repeat these procedures with your left hand on the right foot.

For some it may be easier to use the right hand to work the reflexes on the left foot, and for others to use the right hand to work the right foot. Do whichever is easier for you. *Do not overwork* these pressure points the first few times; just work a few seconds on each reflex, and Nature will do her part in good time.

These sex glands and organs are not only for the purpose of reproducing new life, but play another equally important role, that of regenerating the whole body of which they are a part.

Breast Reflexes

Having placed the sex gland reflexes above the soles of the feet, nature also found it appropriate to place the mammary glands above the soles of the feet. The most effective reflex area for the breasts will

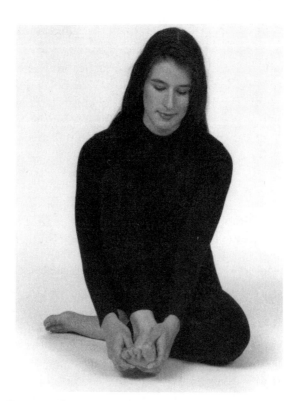

Photo 23. Finger-walk, or use both thumbs, to work the breast reflex area on top of each foot. This technique also stimulates renewed circulation to the chest area, and will encourage healing energy to sore ribs.

be found on top of each foot, on the left foot for left breast, on the right foot for right breast. (See Chart D page 11 and Illustration 3A on page 46.)

Work over the foot from side to side, or up and down the zones. Search for tender spots, and when you find them, reflex the area a little extra. (See Photo 23.)

If you have sore breasts, check for tenderness in all of the endocrine gland reflex areas, as there may be an imbalance of estrogen or progesterone. (Refer to Chart E, page 12.)

Sore Breasts

Women should examine their breasts a couple of days after each monthly period. Lie down and place a small blanket or towel beneath the shoulder of the breast you are going to check. Also place your hand behind your head on the same side of the body; this will help to smooth out the breast so that any lump will be easy to find. Using the hand from opposite side of the body, check breast with index and middle finger, gently working around the outside of breast. Press all the way around and move toward the nipple. If there is a discharge from the nipple, or an unfamiliar lump, you should contact your health care specialist.

Awaken Your Lymph Network

The body has natural disease-fighting antibodies that travel through all parts of the body along with the blood vessels. There are groups of lymph nodes in the groin area, and also in the chest area, the neck and under the arms. Lymph fluid moves within the vessels by way of body motion. Walking is a very good way to get the lymph moving; reflexing the hands and feet is another to awaken the network of lymph.

To stimulate the groups of lymph nodes in the groin and chest area, work reflexes on top of both feet. For this you will use three fingertips from each hand (or if fingers are weak or sore, use the heels of both hands at one time), and stimulate the area above the ankles. Then work your fingers (or heels of both hands) across the top of each foot from ankle to ankle. Read more about the lymphatic system in Chapter 23, page 161. These quick-action workouts are helpful in releasing accumulated fluids and stimulating vital energies throughout the body. They are especially good for improving circulation which will help reduce the swelling that often causes pain.

Reflex Both Feet

To restore all glands to equal efficiency always work the reflexes in both feet because you have glands on both sides of the body.

Work each reflex button only for a few seconds the first few times that you give yourself a reflex workout. Reflexology works in an amazingly short time, if the reflexes are worked as directed here.

This simple reflex therapy can bring women blessed relief from many disorders which may have been troubling them for years. Men also will find relief from what is, in many cases, unsuspected congestion of the gonads (sex glands).

Be persistent and faithful in reflexing these important pressure points, and you will enjoy the results of nature's wonderful healing forces, which are called upon to deal with an unhealthy situation.

SEX GLAND FUNCTIONS

The male sex glands include two testes, the penis, a network of ducts, the prostate gland, and the seminal vesicles. The genital gland has a dual function. Testicles, for instance, externally secrete spermatozoa (reproductive cells), the motile generative element of the semen. But they also internally secrete substances such as the sex hormone testosterone. This hormone affects not only the sexual characteristics, such as muscle mass, growth of penis and body hair, and voice changes, but also affects the whole body, including its mental and personality characteristics, and is essential to one's well-being.

The female sex glands include the ovaries, uterus, fallopian tubes, cervix and the vagina, and the breasts, (breasts are actually mammary glands, which are closely related to sex glands.) Two hormones, estrogen and progesterone, are secreted by the ovaries. Estrogen regulates the growth of body hair, breast development, menstruation, and ovulation. Progesterone gets the uterus ready for pregnancy and contributes to milk production after childbirth. Both hormones coordinate the menstrual cycle. Ovaries influence a woman's appearance, her emotional outlook, and her drives.

No organ can keep its vitality without stimulation by these substances. No wonder these glands (male and female) are so sensitive, since not only are they essential to starting life in a new body (a baby), but they also play a big part in the rejuvenation of our bodies. Never fail to work the reflexes to these valuable glands and organs, no matter how young or old you are. Stagnation is *death*; and circulation is *LIFE!!!*

Reflexes to Prostate Gland

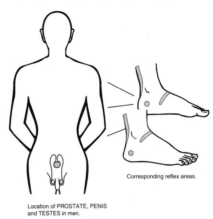

Corresponding reflex areas.

Location of PROSTATE, PENIS and TESTES in men.

The prostate is a male sex gland, and is positioned in front of the rectum, under the bladder, completely encircling the urethra (urinary outlet). It is composed of mucus-secreting glands, essential to effective sperm action.

FUNCTIONS OF THE PROSTATE GLAND

The prostate lies immediately in front of the rectum, so the reflexes for the prostate will be in front of the reflex for the rectum. The prostate neutralizes the acid suspension of sperm, increasing the likelihood of fertilization for reproduction purposes. It is not absolutely essential that the prostate be intact, and because it does not secrete hormones, it is relatively dispensable.

Secretions of the prostate collect in several ducts which emerge into the urethra through a common hillock. Secretion is continuous, with periodic excretion into the urine. You can see what would happen if circulation to this gland is slowed down and congestion results. The flow of secretion from the ducts into the urine would be delayed, and in time the ducts would become swollen and inflamed from obstruction.

If the prostate becomes enlarged due to tightening internal muscles, it will cause the urethra to be partly blocked off. Enlargement of the prostate creates difficulty in voiding the urine, and causes frequent urination, especially during the night. Often there is a burning sensation, and the bladder feels as though it isn't completely empty.

BENEFITS OF PROSTATE REFLEX CONDITIONING

Wholesome and pleasurable sexual relations are healthy for a couple's relationship. Yet many times this enjoyment is disrupted by health challenges. When any section of the prostate is enlarged, the semen has trouble passing through the urethra, causing possible sexual difficulties.

Moreover, when urine cannot pass out of the bladder, it can back up into the kidneys and become contaminated; this disorder will cause other bodily complaints as well as considerable pain.

Don't allow prostate disorders to interfere with your sleep or healthy relationships. There are options to swollen, tight prostate difficulties, such as reflexology which is effective in increasing circulation and balancing the systems of the body.

This gland can cause so much suffering in men, in some cases for years; yet it is so simple to bring it back to health by working the prostate reflexes. I have brought complete relief to every man who came to me with these personal troubles; many times it took only two or three reflex sessions to start the normal circulation returning to the inflamed and enlarged glands. Complications of inflammation or enlargement of the prostate gland just seemed to magically disappear.

SPECIAL PROSTATE REFLEX TECHNIQUES

Get into position to work the reflexes to the prostate, which will be in the same location on both feet. We will use the illustration for reflexing the prostate (refer to Photo 22, page 142). The thumb is pressing on the prostate reflex; notice how it presses specifically in the fleshy part between the ankle and the heel on the inside of the foot. Another technique of working this reflex is to place the index and middle fingers on the fleshy area under the ankle and gently work with a circular pressing motion. Work all around the ankle down to the rectum relfex and back toward the heel.

Continue reflexing down to the heel area, and then work the assistant prostate reflex, which is effective in dealing with these discomforts. To do this use a gentle pinching movement; work up the cords on the back side of the leg (along both sides of the Achilles tendon). If you have the left leg in position, use the right hand for working this reflex. Be sure you reflex both feet.

The reflexes here may be very sore; if so, rotate the ankle a few times in both directions to help stimulate circulation and reduce swelling.

PROSTATE TROUBLE GIVES NO ADVANCE PUBLICITY

Many times prostate trouble starts in young men and advances slowly without their ever being conscious of its increasing danger, until the gland becomes congested enough to cause them discomfort and pain.

I have discovered many congested prostate glands in men who came to me for other complaints. The congestion had not advanced sufficiently to cause any adverse symptoms, so the patients were not aware that it was there. This is so true of many diseases; they creep up on us slowly and secretly until they are well established, and then they strike us suddenly.

This is the wonderful magic of reflexology: it not only helps nature maintain a free-flowing distribution of blood to renew sick and worn-out cells, but it helps send a surge of stimulating, life-giving circulation throughout every cell in the body so that congestion will not have a chance to build up for a sneak attack in the future.

CASES OF PROSTATE HEALING

One elderly man, Mr. B., came to me as a last hope for relief of prostate troubles. He hadn't had a good night's sleep in three months because he had to get up so often to urinate. He had major discomfort from the enlarged gland and was extremely nervous, as this complaint does affect the nervous system.

I was surprised to find a man of his age in such fine health; the only tender place on his feet was the one leading to the prostate. When I remarked about this, he said that otherwise he did enjoy perfect health. The prostate reflexes were extremely tender, and I had to use very little pressure at first. After reflexing only a few minutes he remarked that he felt quite relaxed and that the pressure seemed much less.

When Mr. B. returned for his second session two days later, he was very happy to tell me that he had slept like a baby all night through, didn't have to get up during the night, and felt much better. I noted when I worked the reflexes for the second time that most of the tenderness was gone. I did not see Mr. B again, but his daughter says he is still doing fine. His perfect health condition, other than the congested prostate, probably was a factor in his quick recovery.

How a Stubborn Case of "Prostate" Was Healed

When Mr. F. called my office for an appointment he said he thought his problem was "prostate trouble." I assured him that we had been unbelievably successful working on this condition with reflexology.

I started with Mr. F.'s big toe, seeking a tender spot in the center which would tell me what condition the pituitary gland was in. I found a tremendous response to reflexing in the center of his big toe, as I had expected if the prostate was not functioning properly. Next, I moved on down the foot, pressing and searching for other "messages" that the reflexes could give me pertaining to his condition.

As I worked the reflexes on his feet, Mr. F. told me the symptoms of distress. He was subject to spells of illness if he overworked, or if he ate certain foods such as asparagus, of which he was so fond that he had a large garden full of it. The whole lower region of the abdomen would become sore and "tight" as if everything from his waist down were inflamed. He would became quite ill and have to remain in bed for several days at a time with hardly any food. Doctors had suggested that it might be prostate gland trouble. They had given him treatment for it which had not helped, and as he grew older, each episode seemed more severe.

As I started the reflex application under the ankle bone, I found that the reflexes to the testes were much more tender than the ones to the prostate. When I told him so, he said that when he was quite young, he had been injured by a fall from a horse and that the doctors had had to remove one of the testes, but he had never had any trouble from the other one so far as he could tell.

I found the reflexes to both of the testes so tender that I could barely touch them. The reflex on the left foot was worse than the one on the right; and since the right testis had been removed, the tender reflex to it was an indication of scar tissue. You will find this true in many cases of an operation or injury. The reflexes will always tell you if there is an obstruction or constriction, and even though scar tissue is necessary to mend an operation site, injury, or serious infection, it can develop into a health problem. Sometimes it is necessary to remove it by surgery.

The claim that working these reflexes can dissolve irritating scar tissue may sound like a pretty bold statement, but if doctors were correct in their diagnoses about some of the cases I have worked on, there is ample evidence to show that reflexology does alleviate the distress.

In the case of Mr. F., the reflex to the testis on the left foot was much more tender than the one on the right, indicating that there most probably lay the root of his problem. I did not find any of the other reflexes in either foot nearly so tender as those under the ankles on the outside of the feet. If his real trouble had been from the prostate, then the reflexes on the inner side of the feet would have given the pain signal when pressed.

I concentrated mainly on the reflex to the pituitary in the big toe, and also on the pineal which has its reflex in the big toe, a little to the side of the location of the pituitary. Then I moved on to the adrenal reflexes located in the center of the foot just over the kidney area.

Now, take warning here again—note that I was careful not to work the adrenal reflexes for over ten seconds on each foot for the first few treatments, because they cannot be reflexed without also stimulating the kidney reflexes. For this reason, a few seconds is all that you must use on this area until most of the tenderness is worked out. This should only take three or four reflex applications.

Mr. F. said he felt so much relief and was so relaxed after the first reflex session that he wanted to come back in two days. He came faithfully for two weeks, even though nearly all of his adverse and painful symptoms had vanished after the third workout.

CHAPTER 21

Reflex Relief for Hemorrhoids

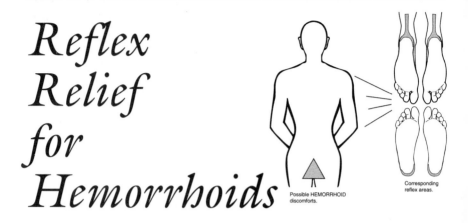

Possible HEMORRHOID discomforts.

Corresponding reflex areas.

Hemorrhoids are nothing more than congested veins (also known as piles). These are actually swollen veins inside or just outside the rectum. They can become so enlarged by inflammation as to protrude, causing great inconvenience, much suffering, and in many cases excessive bleeding.

They are one of the most painful disorders and usually are suffered in silence by those who have them; yet they are one of the quickest to respond with the help of reflexology, at least where pain is concerned.

REFLEX TECHNIQUES

Here we will learn how to use the reflexology method to bring you prompt relief. Lift your leg up into position for reflexing (see Photo 24 for working the reflexes for hemorrhoids). It doesn't make any difference which foot you use first, as both of them will have to be stimulated. You may find one foot more tender than the other when you get started, and, of course, it will be reflexed more. Notice on the above illustration and also on Chart C, the cord up the back of the leg and the edge of the heel is where you find the hemorrhoid reflexes.

If you are using the Reflex Roller here, it will work very nicely on the cord up the back of the leg, but you may have to find the tender reflex on the edge of the heel with the thumb or fingers in a press-and-feel method. If you have the left foot in position, then use the right hand for reflexing as shown in Photo 24. Here you can use a different motion; instead of rolling with the thumb, it is better to press on the bony edge of the heel and press downward toward the heel pad with a firm pulling-down motion. (See illustration 5, page 47.) Or go all the way around the heel, using the thumb on one side and the forefinger on the other side. Use the technique most convenient for you to work with the best amount of pressure.

The tender reflex may only cover the area of a small bean, but you will know it when you press it. That will probably be the reflex to the congested vein in the rectum which is causing all the trouble. Sometimes there is just one sore spot; other times there may be several. You will soon learn where these tender buttons are and be able to find them immediately when irritating symptoms of hemorrhoids start to develop, such as itching or swelling in the rectal area. If you have trouble finding the spot, keep pressing and moving the fingers back and forth, and press in deeper until you do find it. It is there!

For additional help controlling the pain of hemorrhoids, work the reflexes of the digestive system, especially the lower abdominal

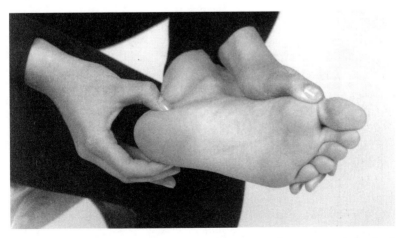

Photo 24. This position is ideal for working the reflexes around the heel to relieve pain of hemorrhoids.

area. Use a pressing motion at the waistline and down along the instep of each foot to the heel; this will cover the lower back and rectal reflex. Continue working back and forth across the heel area to stimulate renewed circulation to the intestine and colon. If your feet have a heavy texture of skin on the heel, you may need to use a reflex tool to reach the necessary reflex areas.

Give some extra attention to the reflexes that correspond to the mid to lower back, to the heart, and also to the liver. (Refer to Charts B and C.) Stimulating these will help reestablish circulation to these very important organs, which in many cases are helper areas for problems associated with hemorrhoids.

Working the Achilles Tendon

Now let's work the cord on the back of the leg, starting just above the heel as shown on Illustration 30a, on page 273. The best way to work this reflex is to put the thumb on one side of the cord and the fingers on the other side and press them up and down from the heel up to where the tendon disappears into the calf of the leg. This area can sometimes be unbearably tender and you will have to start with a "feather touch," increasing the pressure as the tenderness diminishes. Remember, this area contains assistant (or helper) reflexes to all of the lower region of the body, such as the prostate and gonad glands. It also stimulates the lower lumbar region.

Bend the foot as far back as possible, stretching the cord and reflexing it in this position a few moments; then stretch the foot out to the side as far as possible and again work the Achilles tendon. We want this cord to become limber and relaxed, which may take some time to accomplish. The tenderness may be very severe and you will think you can't stand the pain, but the result will be worth the "torture," as some call it. Remember, as the tenderness gradually works out, the condition will improve. The more the pain, the more the inflammation in that area.

Another condition that can cause untold agony is a prolapsed rectum, and as a person gets older, this will probably become worse, protruding more and more. It is very often badly swollen and very much inflamed. The benefits and results from the use of reflexology are almost unbelievable for this serious disorder. Use the same method as for the hemorrhoid and rectum disorders. It is as unique as it is effective. Don't let the simplicity of reflexology deceive you about its importance in healing.

Take Action to Prevent Hemorrhoids

Prevention in the early stages may prevent hemorrhoids, which can be caused by constipation. In order to have effectual bowel movements without troubling your bottom, avoid hard straining. It is important to adjust your diet and eat foods that keep your stools soft, such as plenty of high fiber and vegetable cellulose. Also drink a lot of healthy liquids.

Do not postpone passing waste matter from the large intestine, because the feces lose moisture the longer they remain in the colon, thus making them hard and dry. Then, as you strain to eliminate the hardened feces, veins in the rectum swell and hemorrhoidal development starts.

Other sources of hemorrhoidal irritation are heavy lifting, obesity, allergies, and the lack of exercise. Some hemorrhoids are related to problems of the heart, others to liver damage.

Pregnancy can also contribute to the pain associated with hemorrhoids. When the uterus becomes larger and places pressure on rectal veins, circulation is often slowed down. One very good tip for pregnant women, or for those who are overweight, is to lie on your left side. This takes the pressure off the main vessels that carry blood back and forth to your heart and lungs. With pressure off the veins, circulation improves.

So remember to take the actions necessary to avoid hemorrhoids: adjust your diet to emphasize foods that keep your stools soft; exercise regularly to keep your circulation moving; and use reflexology on the sore reflexes around the heel pads for blessed relief of painful hemorrhoid affliction.

CHAPTER 22

Reflex Areas to the Sciatic Nerve

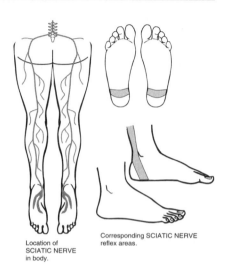

Location of SCIATIC NERVE in body.

Corresponding SCIATIC NERVE reflex areas.

The great sciatic nerve is the largest nerve cord in the body, measuring three-quarters of an inch in width. It passes out of the pelvis and descends along the back part of the thigh to about its lower third where it divides into two large branches. It supplies nearly the whole of the integument of the leg, the muscles of the back of the thigh, and those of the leg and foot.

Inflammation of the sciatic nerve creates intense pain. Many people suffer for years without getting any relief. I believe that I have treated more cases of leg aches than any other malady, and most of them were caused by inflammation of the sciatic nerve.

There can be several reasons for this nerve causing such intense pain: an injury to some other part of the body, an enlarged prostate gland, constipation, and many times a misplacement in the lower spine.

You can readily see the agony that one goes through when inflammation has slowed down the circulation of this large nerve that affects almost the whole lower part of the body. Yet it is so amazingly simple to banish all inflammation in an unbelievably short time by working the reflexes to it.

REFLEX TECHNIQUES

Let us lift the leg into position. Begin with the leg that has the aches and pains. Lift it up into the position for reflexing (see Photo 25 and notice that the Reflex Probe is being used here).

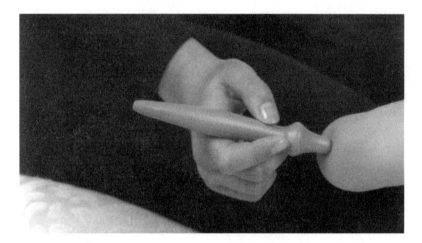

Photo 25. Using the Reflex Probe is an easy and effective technique for working the reflex areas in the heel, where skin tissue is thicker.

It is doubtful that you can reach this particular reflex with the thumb or knuckle unless it is extremely tender; then it would be difficult to reflex with enough pressure to pulverize the crystals causing the congestion. Because the reflex is usually quite deep, take the probe or other self-help tool in your hand and press it into the bottom of the heel, as in the photo. The reflex will be found almost, but not quite, in the center of the heel pad, a little back from the center and toward the inside of the foot (notice position in photo). The way to find the exact spot is to use the press-and-feel method. If you are pressing hard enough, you will know when you find the reflex button because of intense pain.

The treatment is better if it can be done with no covering on the legs, especially silk or rayon. Always work the reflexes on both feet and both legs.

REFLEX LOCATIONS

Now, having found the spot, work it with a deep, rolling motion. At first it may be so tender that it will bring tears to your eyes. Relax the pressure a little until the pain subsides. In many cases, reflexing the end of this great nerve has brought complete relief from leg aches with just one workout. Yours may take several reflex sessions, or the pain could be gone after only one treatment. If it works for others it will work for you, if you follow the directions and use them faithfully. Continue with the reflex workouts until the torture of persistent leg aches stops, and they will if the pains are caused by a congested sciatic nerve. Reflex only a few moments at first.

We have just worked the spot where the sciatic nerve crosses the heel. Now let us move on up to the inner side of the ankle bone where the nerve lies nearest the surface. With the thumb, press above and in back of the ankle. You will probably experience intense pain in this area but not from the sciatic nerve alone. As you can see from Chart C, this covers reflexes to most of the lower extremities of the body. When you are reflexing this area, you are sending the healing forces of nature to all inflamed and congested parts in the lower lumbar region. Work this area with a pressing, rolling motion.

Reflex Area Back of Ankle

Next work the whole area along the Achilles tendon in back of the ankle.

Follow that with a reflex of the entire area above the heel and along the cord at the back of the leg on both sides, as you would for prostate, hemorrhoids, and the lower lumbar region.

Working Up to the Knee Area

Keeping the same position, in back of the ankle, reflex on up the inside of the leg, working up the bone until you come to the knee. You will come across several places that are more tender than others; work these a few seconds, then continue on to the next tender spot. These are like signal buttons buried under the skin. Touch one and it flashes a pain signal telling that there is trouble in the circulation line—so work it out. The Rollo Reflexer may be used for easier stimulation of this area. Work slowly and gently all the way to the knee. The number of sore spots will come as a surprise, especially around the knee area. The reflex should always be gentle, with the self-help tools or fingers pressing in as deeply as the tenderness will permit.

Next do the same progressive reflex work up the outside of the leg, starting at the back of the ankle bone, ending at the knee. This stimulates circulation in the legs, banishes congestion, and brings blessed relief from many leg troubles.

An Additional Reflex from the Back

We will go on to work one more reflex to the sciatic nerve. Reach around to the back a little below the waistline, put your fingers on your spine, about 1 or 2 inches up from your tailbone or end of the spine. Now move the fingers toward the front of the body about the width of the hand where you can feel the movement of the joint of the upper leg. Press in and around this joint with thumb or finger until a severe pain is felt, or at least a sore spot. There again the method must be press-and-feel for the signal button. When it is located, wonders can be accomplished for healing the sciatic nerve by the simple process of pressing on it with the finger, not hard, but holding it as long as the pressure is endurable—like holding in the button on a doorbell.

If you have found the correct position, the sensation will be like that caused by a hot poker being thrust in the joint.

Sciatic pain may be caused by a pinched nerve in the spine. Reflex the whole spine area on the instep of each foot, searching for tenderness. If a sore spot is found here, work it out.

A CASE OF SCIATIC HEALING

Mr. M., a college professor and Naval Reserve officer, came to me with a terrible pain in his heel. He had run the gauntlet of Navy hospitals and private doctors whose only service, he said, was to give him deadening shots in the heel which would last at the most three hours—and the condition was becoming worse. He came to me without any faith, but at the insistence of his wife and neighbors. When I told him I thought I knew what was the matter with him, he seemed quite surprised.

When I pressed into the sciatic nerve reflex in the bottom of his heel, he nearly jumped out of the chair with pain. "That is it!" he said. He was amazed at the almost instant relief, and after only one more reflex session he never had a recurrence of sciatic trouble. If you don't get such gratifying results in three days, remember, persistent effort and a little patience will accomplish the desired results.

Nature Is the Healer

Dear Mrs. Carter:

Nature is the healer of my body. Nature's healing power is much more effective than any "pain pill" made by men, and doesn't cost a dime! I have had several aches and pains in my back and neck over the years and always I would take an aspirin to relieve the pain, but now I am brought instant relief by working the corresponding spine and neck reflex buttons on my feet. My dad is 61 years old and just retired last year. He often complained about the pains and cramps in his legs. I have helped him a great deal by working the sciatic nerve reflexes that you showed me, and now he very seldom complains about his legs; but when he does, I grab a foot. I wish you could see my mom and dad before I started using reflexology on them, so you could see how much they have improved. Thank you for showing me this wonderful technique.

—Mr. E. C.
Texas

CHAPTER 23

How to Stimulate the Lymphatic System

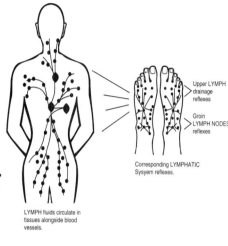

Upper LYMPH drainage reflexes

Groin LYMPH NODES reflexes

Corresponding LYMPHATIC Sysyem reflexes.

LYMPH fluids circulate in tissues alongside blood vessels.

Throughout the body there is an extensive network of fluid, called "lymph," which is vital to life. The lymph system works with the cardiovascular system and has many important functions. Lymph vessels collect fluids which have seeped through the blood vessels' walls and distribute them, or fill tissue, to maintain the body's correct fluid balance.

After the lymph has been cleaned of all waste and impurities, it is returned to the bloodstream via two main lymphatic ducts emptying into subclavian veins. The main lymph channel travels along the spine and circulates through the left side of the body; it then drains into the thoracic duct, which is a large vein on the left side, near the heart. On the right side of the body, just below the neck and shoulder, lymph drains into the right lymphatic duct.

WHAT THE LYMPHATIC SYSTEM DOES

The lymphatic system is one of the body's natural cleaning processes. It has a variety of jobs to do; it works to guard the body from various viruses or diseases. The lymph nodes or glands (enlarged tissue masses in the lymph vessels) are filtering devices for removing dead cells

161

and other foreign matter. They carry away the wastes, bacterias, and viruses from the body's connective tissue. The system also flushes out toxins and excess water, which could otherwise cause congestion and edema.

The lymph nodes near the lungs are black, because lymph from the lungs carries out the dust we breathe. During periods of antibody activity, such as when a finger is infected, the many lymph nodes in the armpit may become swollen and tender as the lymph drains bacteria into this spot.

Or if there is infection on the foot, there may be a swelling of the lymph nodes in the groin of the leg. This indicates that the nodes are doing their work, and the swelling should subside within two weeks.

Nature placed more than 100 of these little seedlike nodes around the tonsils and adenoids, in the neck, under the armpits, down through the center of the body and in the groin area, as a safeguard against infection. Their importance is realized at once, and so is the need to give them proper stimulation.

Lymph Nodes Are Protective in Many Ways

Lymph plays an important role in our immune system. As scavenger cells fight infection and antibodies attack harmful invaders, the fluids clean tissues and filter out bacteria. They filter out and destroy toxins and microorganisms and stop the spread of infections. The spleen and thymus are also made of lymph tissues. The lymphatic system manufactures white blood cells, so if a virus or bacteria enters the body, more white blood cells will be made to fight off and destroy the infection.

Other functions of this system include digesting of fats, conserving nutrients, and, of course, normalizing fluid balance.

Our Second Circulation System

We often refer to the lymphatic system as our supplementary circulation system because it has the plasma containing white blood cells, which help fight off infections. Lymph vessels are everywhere that blood vessels are; its fluids follow outside the bloodstream and inside the soft tissues of the body.

Our blood is pumped by our heart to keep the circulation moving; however, the lymphatic fluid has no pump to circulate it. It is moved by the contraction of our breathing and by body movements, causing pressure against the arteries and muscles which help assist its flow. Circulation of blood and lymph fluid must be maintained to bring renewed oxygen and nutrients to the tissues, as well as help with the removal of any accumulated poisons or built-up toxins.

Physical, mental, and emotional health all depend on the body's circulation of healthy blood and lymphatic fluid. The natural stimulation of reflexology helps improve the circulation of both.

REFLEX TECHNIQUES

There are several techniques that may be used to work the reflexes of the lymph glands. Use the method that is easiest and most natural for you.

Reflex With Your Thumb

Let us now look at Photo 26 for a very effective position of working the reflexes to these many lymph glands.

Notice how the thumb is curled over the top of the foot just above the ankle, where the groin reflex is located. This whole area on top of the foot is to be reflexed, from outside ankle bone, over the top of foot, to inside ankle bone. In Photo 26 we see the thumb being used, curling across the whole area on top of the foot. Use the whole

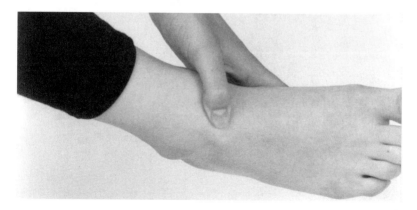

Photo 26. Using your thumb, work over the top of each foot from ankle to ankle to stimulate the reflex areas of the lymph glands in all five zones.

thumb instead of just the end of it in this particular technique, since we are not trying to work a single reflex but many of them. Press and roll the whole thumb over the area using small stationary circles, progressing over the top of the foot.

Reflex With Your Fingers

You may find the simplest way to work these lymph reflexes is to put the left leg up into position on the lap and grasp the inside of the top of the left foot, above the ankle bones, with the left hand, thumb to the inside of the foot. Now, with the fingers curling over the top of the foot, work the whole area, pressing and rolling as you progress back and forth between and just above the ankle bones. Give extra attention wherever you find it tender.

You will find the fingers fit very naturally over the curve of the foot and working this area is easy to do. Also work your fingers over the top of the foot by the toes to stimulate circulation to the neck and throat.

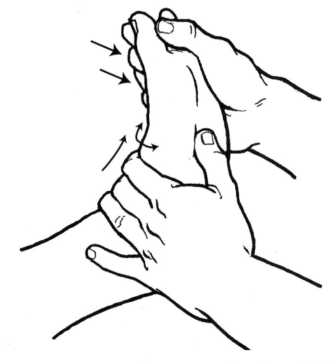

Illustration 17.   Stimulate lymph movement to benefit your health.

Reflex areas for upper lymph drainage are located between the toes, especially between the first and second which correspond to the outside of the neck.

Wrap fingers over the top of the toes and work the webs between them. You can also press-and-roll your thumb on one web at a time. Do the right foot the same way, being sure to always work the reflexes on both feet.

How to Stimulate Lymph Movement with the Heels of Your Hands

To unblock lymph fluid that has become congested, you must get the circulation of fluid moving. Another easy technique is to use the heels of your hands. Start by placing your hands just above the ankles. While the heels of your hands are in a stationary position, continually rotate them forward, keeping contact with foot. Make about seven rotations, then move hands closer together and repeat seven rotations. Using vigorous, circular movements, work over the lymph reflex area from ankle to ankle.

Continue with these various techniques until you have covered the top of the foot. Remember that there are clusters of lymph nodes in several body locations: in the groin (reflexes to groin area are on top, where your foot meets the calf); in the chest and under armpits (reflexes are over top-center and outerside of foot); in the neck, tonsils and adenoids (reflex areas are in the big toe, at the basal joint; work all around the toe, including the top, bottom and sides).

Also benefit upper lymph drainage by working reflexes in between all toes on top of foot.

Walking Stimulates Lymphatic Fluid

This system has no pump (like the heart has), yet it needs to keep its fluid, along with that of the blood vessels, circulating throughout the body. Movement, such as walking, benefits both the cardiovascular system and the lymphatic system. Walk when you can, and when it's not possible, you can just pump your feet to get the fluids moving.

Pumping your feet is simple and fun to do; it takes the place of walking when you can't get out. Bend your feet at the ankles, pointing toes up toward your nose, then point them away from you. If you have a job where you stand or sit most of the time, try this. Or take the opportunity to pump your feet while talking on the phone, when reading or watching TV. This exercise works well anytime.

For an added benefit, raise your feet above the heart, then pump them. When you are lying down, turn onto your back, bend your knees, place one foot flat on the bed and lift the other up above your body and pump it. Or you can lift both feet at the same time. Pump feet forward and backwards, move them in circles to the left, change and move them in circles to the right. Another technique—your wrists have the same reflexes as your ankles; at times it may be easier for you to pump your wrists for additional lymph circulation.

HELP YOUR BODY STRENGTHEN ITS DEFENSE SYSTEMS

Contribute to your own good health by using reflexology to stimulate the vascular and lymphatic systems. The invigorating circulation of blood and lymph throughout the body is absolutely essential to your health; no one can function without it. One of the major roles of the lymph system is to fight off infections. It actually acts as the body's defense program. Antibodies and lymphocytes are made within lymph tissue to filter out disease-causing organisms.

You can activate your healing powers to help fight against the discomfort of seasonal colds, flu, and fatigue. It will be well worth your efforts to work the reflex areas of the heart, vascular, lymph, adenoids, tonsils, thymus, and spleen to help strengthen your body's defense system.

And remember to eat healthy foods to keep your blood rich and strong, as nutrient-laden blood reinforces the disease-fighting powers. Include foods from the basic food groups and include some raw fruits or vegetables every day. Remember, every cell in the body needs a continuous supply of food, water, and oxygen. Proper nutrition and good circulation will help your body build up resistance to those nasty unwanted germs.

CHAPTER 24

How to Condition Reflexes for General Rejuvenation

How old is old? Most people think that their normal life span is "three score years and ten" and if they live beyond the age of 70, they are living on borrowed time.

Would you like to be young again? No, not really! You would not like to part with the knowledge you have gained through the long years of trial and error. But you would like to walk expectantly into the future, to enjoy new experiences, with a revitalized body, wouldn't you? We all would! People say, "If I could just be young again, and know what I know now."

We can do nothing about our chronological age, but we do not have to feel old—or be old—at the age of 70 or even beyond.

According to Dr. Andrew von Salza, a specialist in rejuvenation, "To rejuvenate the body while the mind is saturated with thoughts of senility would not be effective." On the other hand, to expect a healthy mind to produce a healthy body without providing necessary elements conducive to youth would likewise be a fallacy.

Dr. von Salza recommends thinking young to those who feel like senile derelicts. Each person should start a program to prevent senility as a personal task, since at the present time no one is immune to becoming a senile drifter—if he or she lives long enough.

Dr. von Salza goes on to say that quite frequently one becomes a senile derelict overnight—even though senility is not prepared overnight.

"It is prepared," he says, "through years of neglect of the body."

Your body is just as strong as its weakest part. What are your weak points? Tiring easily, slips of memory, wrinkles, difficulty getting up from a chair?

Start to rejuvenate yourself before such signs develop, because when they do develop, your body is sounding an alarm.

Listen for these signals better than you listen to noises in your car. You can buy a new car, but not a new body.

Since time immemorial people have been looking for means of rejuvenation outside of themselves, the search for the "Fountain of Youth," rejuvenation through magic, etc. The only place where there are such possibilities is within yourself.

It is possible to revive glandular vitality in such a measure that the body will be put on the path to reactivate its natural process of rejuvenation—adequate regeneration and growth of cells. Through various therapies the body can be provided with the necessary materials and the will to rebuild itself.

BODY CELLS MUST BE ELECTRICALLY BALANCED

You may have learned in chemistry that the body is made up of a combination of atoms and molecules, and that each atom must have an electrical balance, with the same number of protons (a positive charge) as electrons (a negative charge).

Each body cell is made with a combination of molecules, organelles, and atoms, and must be equally balanced with protons, electrons, and neutrons (neutrons are, as the word implies, neutral). Living in a watery solution, the many types of cells each have a specific job to do and have a highly structured interior.

Reflexing the feet stimulates energy circuits which give Nature a boost. This stimulation encourages a chemical reaction to occur in the living cells; thus the cell's life processes are fueled. Cells of the same kind group together and make tissues; tissues make up organs, such as the heart, lungs, brain, etc. Every second, old cells are dying and new ones are being born; this is how the body works to repair and rebalance itself.

Don't take your body for granted. After all, it is a miracle, an incredible masterpiece, with a brain that helps you learn, and a variety of systems that work together to keep your body going, including your sensory system which helps you enjoy all the wonders of the world around you. So treat yourself to reflexology, Nature's way to balance your health naturally.

ENERGY BALANCE IS ESSENTIAL TO GOOD HEALTH

Reflexology obviously works, as it has been used for several thousands of years. We know that the theory behind reflexology is that reflex areas in the feet and various parts of the body correspond to various organs and glands by way of energy channels. When the appropriate reflex areas are stimulated, vital energy circulates, unblocking any obstructions that may have inhibited its natural flow. When the energy is restored to all systems, balance is normalized, so that the body can heal itself.

Some might ask, what do you mean by normalizing the body's energy balance? And why is it so important? Well, the concept of balance is universal . . . it may be the balance of heaven and earth, of light and dark, or of hot and cold. The Chinese philosophy of yin and yang is a great example of balance; a person with unequal balances of yin or yang cannot be healthy. But when they are rebalanced, the person gets well.

Balanced life energy (like yin and yang) is imperative for a healthy body. All body systems must be balanced with the proper amount of fluid, nutrition, and energy. For this to occur, the body must have good circulation throughout, so that each system can do its specialized job, such as circulating life-giving oxygen and cell-building nutrients, digesting food, or disposing of waste.

Reflexology gets the circulation moving, unblocking obstructions so that the energy can pass through the nerves, helping nature to normalize each of the interior systems. In this way the body is balanced so that everything runs smoothly.

How to Make Reflexology Your Rejuvenator

Reflexology is the scientific method of working the reflexes to stimulate normal circulation which relieves congestion in the various nerve endings. It is a natural and drugless method of stimulating your internal organs, improving blood supply, relieving stress and tension, and promoting deep relaxation.

Most of us do not feel youthful when we are ill or suffering with pain, so the first thing we must do is to help ourselves feel good again.

Many people are not interested in taking care of their health until they start to lose it. Reflexology is a system capable of protecting one's health, preventing illness, and restoring physical and mental energy.

People from all over the world have reported to me over the years that they are living proof of how reflexology has helped improve their health, increased their vitality, and is still keeping them young and strong.

In Great Britain, reflexology is one of the best alternative health modalities. It is used in hospitals, physical therapy centers, and homes to prevent illness and build optimum health. So if you want to improve your health and prevent sickness, you must get to the heart of the problem. First you must eliminate any problems that are causing discomfort; then you can concentrate on the better things in life!

A Basic Reflex Workout

If you suffer pain or illness, search your feet for tenderness. If you find a spot that seems unduly sensitive to the touch, you will want to "work" on this area. Get into a comfortable position, lift your foot and hold it with one hand; with the thumb of the opposite hand press into the sore reflex button. Use a press-and-roll motion to help increase the flow of nerve energy which will keep the body attuned through improved circulation.

Continue this procedure on all sore spots. Repeat every two days until all the soreness is worked out. Working out the sore spots may take several weeks or months, depending on your personal health situation. Remember that the systems in your body work together, and if one part is malfunctioning, the rest of the body will be affected. So the key is to normalize and rebalance the whole body.

Why the Bulgarians Possess Such Great Longevity

In his book, *Health Secrets From Europe*, Dr. Paavo Airola, a Canadian naturopathic doctor and nutritionist, tells us about many of Europe's health clinics and some of the natural health remedies they advise to keep their patients healthfully young.

He tells of Dr. E. M. Hoppe from Sweden, who studied 150 Bulgarian centenarians (100 years or older). His study concentrated on their living and eating habits. Most of them were lacto-vegetarians, eating fresh food from their own gardens, and locally grown and stone-ground whole grains, always freshly ground; they drank milk and ate yogurt from their own sheep. Almost all of them were beekeepers and ate lots of natural honey; they also ate sauerkraut and sunflower seeds regularly. They ate very small amounts of meat (only 5 of the 150 questioned ate meat regularly). Most worked hard on farms and were extremely poor, so they did not overeat. These people had no stress in their lives, and followed nature's rhythm in sleeping, eating, and working.

By this study, we know that wholesome natural foods, stress-free living, and hard work (keeping the circulation moving) are scientifically proven factors in preventing premature aging and prolonging life!

Dr. Airola tells us that, according to one census, there are more centenarians in Bulgaria than in any other civilized country: 1,600 centenarians to every million persons, compared with 9 centenarians to every million persons in the United States.

Fifteen Steps to Improve Your Health and Restore Youthfulness

1. Use reflexology on a regular basis to relieve stress and tension from your body.

2. Do as the centenarian Bulgarians do and help yourself prevent premature aging by eating natural foods, exercising, and getting plenty of stress-free rest.

3. Reverse the aging process by using reflexology to reactivate the organs of elimination, especially the liver and kidneys.

4. Drink a lot of pure water to improve digestive efficiency and flush out toxins, prevent constipation, and help hydrate your skin and hair; water will also give you added energy.

5. Increase your immune power by eating raw foods and juices. Eat fresh or frozen foods for a generous supply of enzymes (which are known as miracle health builders) or take vitamin and mineral supplements every day. Grains and seeds are also rich sources of natural enzymes. Raw foods will help regenerate your skin tissues, so that they will stay smooth and supple. (These enzymes benefit tissues of glands and organs on the inside of the body, as well as the skin on the outside of the body.)

6. Reflexing the top of your feet will invigorate your lymphatic system, which will boost your immune power to fight infection and keep you feeling young and healthy.

7. Reflexology and deep breathing are a good combination to bring renewed oxygen to your cells, keeping them activated, and helping free you from aging at a rapid rate.

8. Use the Deluxe-Foot-Roller or Magic Reflexer to stimulate reflexes and send a flow of energized electrical life force through your whole body to wake up cells and protect you against premature aging.

9. Look and feel younger with an optimistic outlook. Be cheerful and remember to smile; it stimulates your immune system and actually releases adrenaline, to renew your vitality.

10. Remember to take the time for things you enjoy in life, such as your hobbies, reading, and listening to music. Doing the things you enjoy helps your mind stay refreshingly active and healthy.

11. One of the keys to feeling youthful and dynamic is happiness, so observe the wonderful world around you. Take time to enjoy pretty colors, flowers, animals, and your friendships.

12. Rejuvenate yourself with love and romance. Another key to feeling younger is acting younger. Occasionally you must let the worries go and make the most of life's little pleasures.

13. Get plenty of exercise; walking is **excellent** (use reflex stimulation if you can't walk).

14. Reflexology helps improve the blood supply. In conjunction with a diet of simple, natural nutrition, it will help balance blood pressure and may prevent heart problems.

15. Reflexology, meditation, visualization, and frequent rest breaks will help you enjoy the benefits of a stress-free life. Reduced stress will help you feel younger and most likely will help you live longer!

You can win the war against premature aging! Use reflexology to release congestion that inhibits energy flow and renews healthful circulation. Improve your diet with health-building foods, and get proper exercise.

With the Help of Reflexology, Life Begins at Seventy-Eight

Dear Mildred Carter,

About two and one-half years ago I was looking forward only to the life of an invalid, and my health was getting worse every day. New pains and health problems kept popping up and I had tried so hard to keep going, since there was no one to look out for me if I became bedridden.

A friend of mine came by and brought a copy of your book on Foot Reflexology. I started trying to apply the information gained through it to my own troubles. What made it so difficult was that I could only reach my right foot, since the full length of the left leg, including the hip and pelvis, had all been broken six years before from a fall on an ice slick. Doctors had decided that my heart was in too bad a condition to set and patch up the broken thigh, knee, and ankle. And that side had withered and shortened a full five inches, and could in no way be leaned down to, or bent without excruciating pain.

I studied your book carefully, memorized a lot of it, and started to work on the right foot. About that time I read where you said to never work on just one side. However, I had been working on just one foot for three days, and I was beginning to feel better. You had mentioned that one could also be helped by hand reflexology, and though I hadn't the slightest notion how to find the reflexes in my hands, I started searching out the tender or sore spots in them, the same as you had said to do in the feet. One by one, day by day, I kept working and pressing on the sore points in both hands and one foot. IT WORKED!!!!!

I was almost seventy-six then. Now I'm seventy-eight past, and still using your reflexology instructions; I have them memorized. The headaches I have had almost daily since age 23 only come once or twice a year instead of every day. Stomach trouble and indigestion are gone, arthritis is fast disappearing, and except for losing the use of my left leg, I feel better than I did twenty years ago. THANK YOU for letting the World know about this. Life begins at seventy-eight! Thanks,

—B. L.

A Case of "Hot Flashes" Healed

Mrs. M. called to ask if there was anything that I could do for hot flashes. They were so bad that she often had to go to bed. The shots the doctors gave her lasted only a few hours and sometimes did not even bring relief. She was desperate because she had to work to support her family.

Since reflexology stimulates the circulation of every gland in the body, I told her to come and see what results we would get. Mrs. M. felt better in the first few minutes of working the reflexes. When she came for her second reflex session two days later, she was elated. She had gone home and slept like a baby the whole night after the reflex workout; she had been free of hot flashes for two days and was just beginning to feel light ones starting again. She felt a new surge of energy, a spiritual uplift, a new zest for life. She did not need very many reflex sessions to balance her system, and as long as I knew her the symptoms never returned. This is worth careful consideration.

How the Reflexes Worked to Rejuvenate

By working the reflex to Mrs. M.'s endocrine glands, especially the ovaries, I stimulated a normal production of the hormone estrogen. Her natural body rebuilding process had started to slow down. With reflexology I put the process in reverse by working the reflex to the pituitary gland and relieving congestion, to place those hormones back into circulation. I also stimulated the endocrine glands so that they were able to produce and pour into the cellulary system certain substances which regulate the metabolic processes, growth, and morphology of cells. This we must have to keep young.

So long as the rebuilding of cells is adequate, the organism is young. As soon as this rebuilding process starts to slow down, the organism is getting old—and so are you!

A CASE OF SENILITY HELPED

I also rejuvenated my ailing, senile, 85-year-old mother, treating her myself after taking her out of the hospital. She became a pleasant, happy companion for many years.

One of her favorite reflexes for relieving body tension was the foot twist. Let us learn to give the stimulating reflex that will bring relaxation to the entire body (see Photo 27.)

Take the foot up on the lap as shown in the photo. Take the end of the foot in the opposite hand and, with a rolling motion, twist the

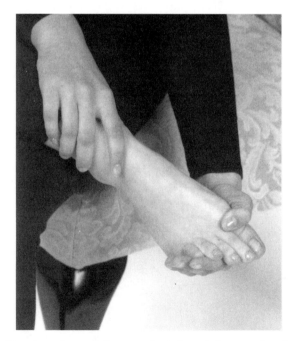

Photo 27. Gently twist each foot to the left and then to the right to relieve body tension.

whole foot. Roll the foot in as large a circle as you can. Don't force it; just roll it gently around and around, twisting as you roll (note Photo 27). This will relax the tension of the whole body, as if someone were giving you a body massage. If the foot seems stiff and tense, then your body is in a like condition. After you have limbered the foot up a bit, reverse the rolling procedure and roll it in the opposite direction; then change feet, using the same procedure. I find it is good to start out with a few seconds of this relaxing technique at the beginning of the treatments, and then use it again at the end of the session.

I have proved this scientific method of healing beyond a doubt in my experience. Try it on yourself and *feel* the beneficial results.

How Reflexology Helps Improve Health of All Glands

Every cell in the human body is capable of being energized by the substances emitted from the endocrine glands, the seven centers of vital force which act as electrical battery storages for the purpose of constantly recreating life.

Therefore, a major requisite for a perfect body is to have the cellular tissue mineralized, vitaminized, and hence ionized to receive these emanations. Minerals and vitamins must be absorbed into the bloodstream; the vitamins bring the otherwise dead minerals to life.

THE GLANDS AS "WATCHDOGS OF THE BODY"

The glands have been aptly termed the "watchdogs of the body." They trap the necessary nutriments, and, in conjunction with their internal secretions, form them into powerful crystallization (much as the essences of flowers are mixed with the internal secretions of the bees to be converted into honey).

These crystallizations are named hormones which influence all the activities of life. An example would be a deficiency of the thyroid secretion, which would prevent the natural growth of the body and interfere with the rhythmical functioning of the heart.

A deficiency of the sex hormone would cause sterility and other sex maladjustments, and since there is a close affinity between the complete circle of glands, it would be liable to affect the whole behavior of the person thus afflicted.

The seven endocrine glands are known as the body's main energy centers, or control centers. Each of these glands is a special point of vital life energy, and is a link between brain and body. To keep these glands charged and vitalized is to keep the mind and body healthy.

It has been claimed that the hormones send out radio-electric emanations which have been generated in the glandular powerhouses. The radiant waves travel along the cerebro-nervous system, which, when it is tuned to a high state of efficiency, broadcasts waves of energy to the most remote cell in the body. When the waves are not powerful enough, millions of cells are left dormant or stagnant. This is the start of disease, for when too many cells die, the body is reduced to a state of autointoxication.

What Tiredness Indicates

Actually, a feeling of tiredness is an announcement that the generators of the electric charges are not functioning at optimal efficiency. This indicates that the endocrine glands are underactive and are not sufficiently distributing their chemical instructions (hormones) into the bloodstream. Reflexology stimulates the energy needed to rebalance these hormones.

Tiredness also may reveal that there is either a mineral or a vitamin deficiency in the bloodstream. Stimulating the reflexes to all endocrine glands will recharge important control centers, encouraging the chemical messengers (hormones) to balance the body's use of food, oxygen, and various nutrients.

Reflexology will touch off the spark needed to rebalance all these glands. They, in turn, promote proper functioning of every other part of the body, help to regulate blood pressure, heartbeat, produce needed insulin and adrenaline, and supply the body with extra energy.

THE ENDOCRINE GLANDS MUST WORK IN PERFECT HARMONY

Let us look, then, at these watchdogs, the endocrine glands. These are often identified as the ductless glands because most of them do not have ducts, and secrete their hormones directly into the bloodstream.

The endocrine system is comprised of the pituitary, hypothalamus, and pineal glands, situated in the cavity of the skull; the thyroid and parathyroids near the larynx at the base of the neck; the thymus which lies in the chest above the heart; the pancreas which is located in the mid-stomach area; a pair of adrenals placed atop the kidneys like two little hoods; and the gonads, the sex glands.

These so-called ductless glands cooperate in determining the forms of our bodies and the workings of our minds. They are all closely interrelated and supplement and depend on each other.

Every individual owes his or her development and well-being to the normal functioning of these glands. The minute secretions called hormones sent into the bloodstream by these glands are responsible for the difference between a genius and an imbecile, between a little person and a giant, between a person who is happy and one who is cheerless.

The potency of the endocrine glands is beyond comprehension. They control our activity, energy, stabilization, radiance, mobility, and organization of life processes.

They are also the main glands that the reflexes will stimulate to normal performance, and that herbs nourish with their wealth of vitamins and minerals.

It is very likely that many of the synthetic medicines put into the blood are responsible for the malfunctioning of one or the other of these glands, and they do have to work in perfect harmony with each other; otherwise, all sorts of ailments will occur in the body.

Hormones Control the Body's Processes

Hormones are like little messengers which travel from the hypothalamus to the pituitary gland. From there they move into the bloodstream, stimulating other endocrine glands and telling them each to produce their own hormones. These hormones travel to receptors inside the cells with their message.

Hormones have a lot of extraordinary jobs to do, such as to regulate the mineral and water balance of the body, to regulate nutrients that are absorbed into the cells, and work some hormones to control levels of blood sugar (insulin). Other hormones affect growth rate and metabolism, blood pressure, and the nervous system.

There are even hormones that help when giving birth. These designated hormones carry a message to the uterus, telling it to contract during childbirth. Then they signal tissues which activate the production of breast milk.

THE REWARDS OF HARMONIZING YOUR GLAND ACTIVITIES

Learning to live so that the endocrine glands harmonize will, in turn, enable you to live with a sound body and vibrant health. As you reflex these important control centers you will be helping to balance the body's natural hormone processes. As these glands are harmonized they will be able to perform their major tasks and coordinate the activity of your other systems. As your body conforms, you will find your illnesses inclined to vanish. The secret is to stimulate each of them in every natural way available.

Pituitary Gland

The diagram of the endocrine glands (Chart E) shows one of the most important glands, the pituitary, located at the base of the brain just at the midpoint of the head, as though carefully hidden in the safest and most inaccessible place—and well it should be, as it is vastly needed. Although it is only about 1/40th of an ounce, it has the biggest job to do, that of keeping the other glands in harmony with each other. Its task could be compared to that of first violin, on which a great orchestra depends!

Together with the hypothalamus which regulates hormone production, the pituitary gland, which produces "master" hormones, controls the inner mobility and agility of the system, promoting the proper growth of the body, glands, and organs, including female menstrual cycle, sexual development, and sexual drive. It maintains the efficiency of the various structures and prevents the excessive accumulation of fat. A relaxed, harmonious, and happy person, without complexes and frustrations, is sure to possess a normal, healthy, and active pituitary gland.

Remember the reflexes for the pituitary are located in the center of each big toe.

It is known that the pituitary gland secretes hormones into the bloodstream. It actually is divided into two parts, or rather, two separate glands, the rear section is the posterior lobe and the forward portion the anterior lobe. Both lobes produce polypeptide hormones. The anterior lobe produces at least six hormones that have been definitely isolated as pure, or nearly pure, substances. The existence of several other hormones is suspected.

Of the various hormones, one has been found to have the function of stimulating the thyroid gland: thyroid-stimulating hormone (TSH). Another stimulates the function of the testes and ovaries; it is called follicle-stimulating hormone (FSH). Thus, it can be seen how important it is to keep the pituitary stimulated with reflexology and in perfect working order.

The Hypothalamus

Your hypothalamus is the link between your endocrine system and autonomic nervous system. It is located in the brain, just above the pituitary gland and is connected to the spinal cord by way of many nerves. It controls pituitary secretions and regulates the production of hormones, as well as many body functions including sleep, wakefulness, thirst, and hunger. When you reach the correct reflex of the pituitary gland, you are also on that of the hypothalamus.

Pineal Gland

Note that the pineal gland lies quite close to the pituitary with the same treatments generally used for it. Its reflexes are a little to the side of the center of the big toe.

It has been established that a pathological condition of this gland strongly influences the sex glands, causing premature development of the entire system.

It acts with the body as a sort of organizer, or harmonizer, controlling the development of the glands and keeping them in proper range. The pineal gland's normal activity keeps the functions of the endocrine system harmonious and effective.

Even smaller than the pituitary, this gland is important to one's well-being.

Thyroid Gland

The thyroid is a small hormone-producing gland in the front of the neck. It is a soft mass of yellowish-red, glandular tissue about 2 inches high and slightly more than 2 inches wide, weighing an ounce or less. It exists in two lobes, one on either side of the windpipe with a narrow, connecting band running in front of the windpipe just at the bottom of what is commonly known as the Adam's apple (see Chart E).

The thyroid produces the hormone thyroxine, an iodine-protein compound, and tri-iodothyronine. These are made up of carbon, hydrogen, nitrogen, and oxygen.

Exactly what is the importance of the thyroid gland, and what is its influence on the body?

The degree of thyroid activity makes one either alert or dull, quick or slow, animated or depressed, mentally keen or apathetic. It is also responsible for the inner activity of one's system, preventing the retention of water, sluggishness of the tissues, and densification of the bones.

The growth rate of cells depends on the hormones produced by the thyroid, as it controls the rate at which food and oxygen are converted into heat and energy in all cells.

Proper development of, and functioning of, the sex organs also depends upon the healthy and normal functioning of the thyroid.

An enlargement of this gland is called a goiter. Since we now know of iodine's beneficial effect, this trouble is seldom encountered any more.

The reflex to the thyroid is down from the big toe, at the basal joint and to the center of the foot ever so little. Work all around the base of the big toe. Reflex of the entire area is important, from just under the toe down to the inner edge of the foot.

Any seeming difficulty with the thyroid is quite possibly caused by a malfunctioning of the pituitary which is affecting this gland.

Parathyroid Glands

Beneath the surface of the thyroid gland are four flattened scraps of pinkish-reddish tissue, each about one-third of an inch long. Two are on either side of the windpipe, one of each pair near the top of the thyroid and one near the bottom. These are the parathyroid glands, shown in Chart E.

These glands influence the stability within the body, the maintenance of its metabolic equilibrium, by controlling the distribution and activity of calcium and phosphorus in the system.

Calcium is essential not only to bones and teeth but to blood coagulation, and to the proper working of nerve and muscle. To do its work properly, calcium must remain within a narrow range of concentration. Should it rise too high or drop too low, the entire ion balance of the blood is upset. When the calcium count is high, it causes weak muscle tone and kidney stones. When it is too low the body must draw it from the bones, leaving them brittle. Neither nerves nor muscles can work without proper balance; and the body, through a failure in organization, dies. It is the proper functioning of the parathyroid gland which keeps this from happening. Poise and tranquility are the results of the normal functioning of these glands.

The reflexes will be the same as for the thyroid, except that there appears to be a need for *deeper* stimulation. Press slightly harder in the area of the thyroid, working back behind it, careful not to bruise the tissue or capillaries.

Thymus Gland

We are born with the thymus gland lying in the upper chest in front of the lungs and above the heart, just below the thyroid gland, as shown in Chart E. It influences the activities of the spleen and lymph glands and helps produce a white blood cell that fights off infections.

In children the thymus is soft and pink, with mazy lobes. It is fairly large, weighing as much as 40 grams or 1½ ounces.

As puberty is reached, the gland diminishes in importance as well as in size.

To reflex the thymus gland, work the area of the foot just below the thyroid reflex.

As long as the other endocrine glands are kept in harmony with each other, there is no occasion to be overly concerned about the thymus.

Adrenal Glands

The adrenal glands, small caps astride the kidneys, influence all our activities, our vigor, courage, and passions. They promote the inner drive to action, keen perception, and untiring activity.

They are sometimes referred to as the "fight or flight" glands, or the body's natural alarm system. Under pressure of strong emotion, the gland releases two hormones, adrenalin and noradrenalin, which have an immediate and profound effect on the machinery of the body by mobilizing its resources for a state of emergency. Heartbeat is accelerated, circulation is increased, blood sugar level rises. You breathe in more air and suddenly you have a rush of energy. The noradrenalin hormone stimulates fear, while the adrenalin hormone tends to make one angry and ready to fight.

It is a fairly well-established fact that the timid, introverted, neurotic type of person possesses adrenal glands that are not producing a sufficient amount of adrenalin, and too large an amount of noradrenalin. This results, it is said, from insufficient support, causing degeneration of the glands coupled partly with disturbances within the blood sugar-regulating mechanism.

Now the pituitary gland must help, as both these glands accomplish their functions in controlling the blood-sugar level in this way. When the blood-sugar level starts to dip below normal limits, the pituitary secretes what is called ACTH (adrenocorticotropic hormone) into the blood. This is picked up by the adrenal gland and stimulates it into secreting cortisone and cortin into the blood. These adrenal hormones, in turn, cause the liver, as well as the body's muscles, to give up some of their stored body sugar. Through the action of the hormone the pancreas produces, glucagon is released and changed into soluble glucose, the blood form of sugar. This process takes place until the blood's sugar is up to a normal level.

If the adrenal glands were permitted to lose their efficiency or become impaired in function, the body would be in for serious trouble, and probably the mind as well, since the brain must have a constant supply of sugar at all times or it will become critically damaged.

It must be kept in mind that the glands make this blood sugar out of the foods eaten. Commercial sugars are not referred to here, but rather the natural sugars such as those found in fruits and vegetables.

Here again, medical science has many questions still unanswered about the entire physical-chemical spectrum. However, in treating any and all parts of the body with nature's remedies, there is no risk from repercussions of experimental backfiring.

The adrenal glands appear to have considerably more need for vitamin C and the B complex group, as well as vitamin A.

Reflexes to the adrenals will be almost the same as for the kidneys, found almost in the center of each foot just a bit up from the waistline of the foot. (See Chart E.) If using the Reflex Roller be sure not to overdo the first week, since the adrenals cannot be worked without stimulating the reflex to the kidneys, which can be overworked too much at first.

The Pancreas

The pancreas is a large gland located behind the stomach and measures from 6 to 8 inches in length. It is actually two organs in one. It produces pancreatic juice and manufactures hormones. It has a dual role, acting both as an endocrine and an exocrine organ.

Pancreatic juice is a fluid containing a mixture of digestive enzymes which come from the nonendocrine cells and help with digestion. Enzymes are secreted into the small intestine to help break foods down into chemicals for the body to use.

Pancreatic juice is essential to many food conversions: of consumed starch into maltose, a type of sugar; of fats into fatty acids and glycerol; of proteins into amino acids. These are then to be reassembled into the specific types of proteins or tissues as needed by the body for growth and repair.

This important endocrine gland produces several hormones, most common of which are insulin and glucagon. Its secretion of insulin is widely recognized as being necessary for turning sugar into the production of energy. Insulin reduces the amount of sugar in the blood by moving it into cells so they can utilize glucose for energy. When there is not enough sugar in the blood, then glucagon is secreted to balance this action. This hormone helps the liver to release sugar into the bloodstream, thus raising the level of sugar in the blood.

This major balancing mechanism is important, especially if you haven't eaten for several hours. Without a healthy pancreas, your tissues, muscles, and brain would all be threatened with a decreasing amount of the very important glucose.

The pancreas is an unusually sensitive organ and its slightest impairment will alter the chemistry of the body which will then be subject to particularly distressing fluctuations. It must function perfectly or the result is diabetes. Fat-consuming nations and peoples of the world seem to suffer the most from diabetes. It has also been found that synthetic corn syrup or corn sugar induces diabetes in test animals. One specific needs of the pancreas that is now known, other than an ordinary healthy diet, is the mineral zinc, which seems to be much less than normal in this gland when diabetes is present.

To keep the pancreas in functioning, healthy condition, be sure to send it life-giving energy by working its reflex. It lies horizontally behind the stomach and in between the kidneys and adrenals. It should get its proper share of stimulation when using the Reflex Roller. But if there is diabetes, beware of overstimulating this particular spot at first. Watch insulin intake, as stimulation to the pancreas can accelerate the production of insulin naturally and it is possible you will not need to take as much. In fact, one diabetic said that he had to cut down over half of his intake of insulin after the second reflex session and he had been taking it for over 20 years!

Gonads

As has been stated, the gonads are the sex glands: ovaries in the female, testes in the male. (See Chart E.)

These glands produce the sex hormones. There is one gland besides the gonads which produces sex hormones, and that is the adrenal gland or cortex. Sparkling eyes, luminosity, self-reliance, and self-assurance are all signs that the gonads are functioning properly. Their hormones create inner warmth in the system, preventing tendencies for inflexibility. They are responsible for the ability to attract others and retain affection. They make our personalities radiant and magnetic.

There is a close relationship between the pituitary and the gonads. Indeed, a failure of the pituitary gland can act the same as a castration or ovariotomy.

An undersecretion of the pituitary in the young can result in very short stature, such as in the case of a little person. An excess of growth hormone, on the other hand, can lead to gigantism, to gross obesity, and to arrested sexual development. Basketball players and members of certain African tribes are not giants; they are simply tall people, with a normal inherited trait.

Endocrine Glands Are Like Little Giants

The endocrine glands are very small and all together weigh only about five ounces. Yet they control many vital body processes. Their secret is in the extraordinary power of the hormones they secrete.

Some of the endocrine glands produce cortisone and other needed substances, many of them probably yet unknown to science.

Researchers keep finding new hormones, and now know of over 100. We still don't know all there is to know about the needs of the body, but when it becomes ill, then we do know that someplace some gland is not supplying something that the body needs to maintain it in perfect working order.

But when we stimulate these glands back into their normal, healthy condition by working their reflexes, naturally they will start producing the life-giving substances which the body has been missing. As the glands return to normal functioning, so will the body return to normal health.

So start working on the closest thing to nature for a natural and sure healing—your feet!

Study Chart E on the endocrine glands and work the reflexes to all of them every other day for the first two weeks; while you are stimulating them, don't neglect the other reflexes that are there in each foot. Remember, when one instrument is out of tune in the orchestra, it throws the rest of the instruments off and we have a song of discord. Your body must be in harmony to give you the perfect health that is your right as long as you live. Every truly healthy person should experience a feeling of exuberance and well-being all day through and be able to fall into a deep, painless sleep at night.

Is this the way you feel? If it isn't, then you are not enjoying the health that nature intended you to have when you were born. All you have to do is TRY! Seek for health by starting on the road to health nature's way.

I presume that you have one of your feet up into position for reflexing. Let us start with the big toe and give it a thorough going over, especially in the center where the reflex to the pituitary gland lies. Then work on each toe and under each one, pressing in with a rolling circular motion. When you find an extremely tender spot be sure to give it a good workout, and then later return to it and work it again, as this soreness indicates trouble in the body. Never forget that although reflexology makes the feet feel like new, our main concern is the healing of the body.

After you have worked over each toe and around it, move on down to the thyroid reflex just under the bone of the big toe, and work it well, pressing in deeply so as to reach the parathyroids' reflexes. These are very important little glands, little but mighty, and you may have to use the Reflex Probe, or a like self-help tool, to reach them. They are deeper than the thyroid and thus harder to reach. After the thyroids, move the fingers on to the adrenal gland reflex in the center of the foot and work it, and then on to the sex glands under the ankles.

Now go back and cover the whole foot, conditioning all of the rest of the reflexes. Always attend to tender spots in the feet. Keep in mind if there is tenderness in the foot there is trouble in the body; so work it out, even if you are not sure what part of the body it goes to. A tender reflex is telling you something is wrong with the corresponding area of the body by giving pain sensations when you press in on it.

Don't neglect any part of the foot. When you have reflexed one foot thoroughly, put it down and pick up the other foot, giving it the same treatment that you have just given this one; thus you will be helping nature to do the healing.

Let's Keep Our Health Naturally

Dear Ms. Carter,

I want to tell you how grateful I am for your wonderful books. I speak about your books to everyone that I know or meet and I have great faith in reflexology. I hope to see the day when operations, drugs and medicines of all sorts will vanish, thus leaving room for the natural God-given way to gain back good health. Then we can keep our health naturally. Thanks again. May God Bless You!

—M.R.

Dr. George Starr White, M.D., who was very involved with using natural methods of healing, including zone therapy, and finding new safeguards to help fight disease, seemed to have also had a good sense of humor. In one of his lectures he was quoted as saying, "Methinks we should reverse the engines and adopt the Chinese plan, namely, that the customer pay the doctor for keeping him well, and not pay when he is not well."

CASE HISTORIES OF ARTHRITIS HEALED

There are so many who have been helped by working the reflexes for arthritis that I could write a book telling you about them. Let me tell you of just two people who came to me.

A man so crippled with arthritis that he could hardly walk was brought to me by his wife. He had to lean on her for support and then was only barely able to hobble into my office. I helped him into the chair and removed his shoes and socks. His poor feet were so curled and misshapen that it was hard to tell where any certain reflex would be located in them. His hands were in the same condition, with the fingers twisted into the palms of the hands. His face was drawn with pain and his eyes had the hopeless look of one who has suffered excruciating agony with no promise of relief.

He had earned his livelihood as a carpenter and now was unable to work and support his family. His wife's employment didn't cover all their expenses and they had to eventually go on welfare, which hurt his pride. The worry only added to his troubles, because stress of any kind seems to add fuel to the fire, as they say, for any arthritis sufferer.

The doctors gave him no hope of relief from this terrible malady and they had spent all of their savings on his doctors and medication. Luckily at that time the welfare agency recognized reflexology as a healing agent and paid for the reflex sessions. Even though I would have given him the treatments anyway, I have found that many people are too proud to accept.

It was almost impossible to locate any certain reflex in his misshapen feet. They were very tender and I had to work very slowly and gently in under the twisted bones. As I worked, the feet seemed to become more relaxed. Pain and worry cause a lot of undue tension on muscles and that occasionally helps to pull the affected areas more out of shape than the arthritis itself. In his case I worked on the hands, too, giving just a few minutes to each foot and each hand.

After a few sessions his hands and feet started to improve. He said that the pain had been so relieved after the first treatment that he had slept the whole night through for the first time in months.

Of course, we know what wonders reflexology does in restoring the normal functions of the body, and in many cases the feeling of renewed hope has much to do with a rapid recovery. In releasing tensions and worry from the mind, the body has a chance to relax and start its way back to normal functioning as nature intended it to.

It wasn't long after he first came to me that his hands and feet began to uncurl and straighten out like the petals of flowers. It was wonderful to watch him improve so rapidly. He was soon able to use his hammer once more and walk naturally on his feet again. You can imagine how elated and thankful he and his wife were. Nature works in wondrous ways if we just know how to give her a chance to rebuild our bodies. Yes, nature knows what to do; after all, how were our bodies built in the first place?

The next case history is of a very wealthy lady who had such severe arthritis that she finally had to use a wheelchair to see me. She was very lucky that she had a husband who devoted his time and money to her every need. He had taken his wife to any doctor who promised any relief at all for her. She had had the most expensive medication money could buy, but when we become ill we are helpless in nature's hands and sometimes all the money in the world cannot buy what nature gives freely.

This lady's knees and ankles were swollen beyond belief. She suffered excruciating agony 24 hours a day, and her devoted husband's face was drawn with pain and worry in his suffering for her. Sometimes we suffer more for a loved one than we do for our own physical pain.

One might have thought her case was hopeless upon seeing the inflamed, swollen joints of this lovely woman as she was wheeled into the office. But as long as people have hope there is always a chance, and if they keep searching they will find a way, nature's way, usually after all other methods have been tried and have failed.

Did she respond to the reflexology treatments? It was like watching a miracle unfold before your eyes to see her rapid recovery after a few weeks of reflexology. Today she is free of pain, and to see her walking down the street in her fancy dress shoes, one would never think that such a very short time ago she was an invalid, wracked with pain.

If reflexology can do this for others, it can do it for you. Keep up your hope and don't get discouraged. Remember, you took a long time to get into the condition that you are in now, so how can you expect nature to completely cure you in a few days or even weeks? The symptoms of arthritis have a bad habit of getting better for a while and raising people's hopes, then letting them down by flooding back with all of the old miseries. In the reflexology sessions, I notice that this surging back and forth of the disease is much less than with other types of treatments, and the improvements seem to be more steady. But if it doesn't happen to you, don't give up! Remember, a tree doesn't grow in a day; patience will prevail.

CHAPTER 26

How to Overcome Stress and Fatigue the Natural Way

Chronic fatigue is the curse of our modern age. In this day of increased leisure and labor-saving gadgets, everyone crowds his or her allotted 24 hours with hectic activity, which results in both physical and mental exhaustion. Many doctors report that their patients complain of "being tired," even when they are unable to find any medical reason for it. Through reflexology, however, fatigue can be relieved quickly and easily at any time, anywhere, by everyone. Let us look at a few typical cases of average people in routine situations.

ALL IN A DAY'S WORK

Let's suppose that you have been rushed all day. You experienced a hectic day at work, stopped at the bank, the market, the florist, and now you are cleaning and dusting and preparing a gourmet dinner for invited guests. As the hour approaches for their arrival, you suddenly feel "beat" and have no energy or enthusiasm left for serving and entertaining. You think, "If there only were some kind of magic tonic to give me an instant pickup!" Well, you do have one, right there on the bottom of your feet.

How to Restore Your Energy With a Reflexology Workout

The Pituitary

Sit down in the nearest chair and kick off your shoes. Lift one foot up into position (either one will do). Now give the center of your big toe a quick workout, remembering to press deeply enough to touch the reflex to the pituitary gland. Then move on down to the thyroid reflex, which is just under the bone of the big toe. If you remember the charts, you will know just which reflexes to work. If you don't, refer to them for best results.

The Adrenals

Next, move your thumb toward the center of the sole to find the reflexes to the adrenal glands. These are the quick-energy glands for the magic tonic you need right *now*. They boost vigor and promote your inner drive to action, giving you unflagging energy. Rotate your thumb, or a tool, on the reflex for about 30 seconds only—remember, you are looking for *a fast pickup* and not a general health treatment. You will feel an immediate recharging of your worn-down body batteries.

Sex Glands

The gonads, or sex glands, are also important in depleting our energies. As I stated in the chapter on glands, the adrenal glands also produce sex hormones. It is from these hormones that you get sparkling eyes and self-reliance, and they make for a radiant and magnetic personality. So, continue with the workout by moving your fingers to the ankle area and stimulate the reflexes, which lie just under the ankle bones on the outside of the foot, for about 15 seconds. Work this area with a slight circular motion, change to the other foot and work it the same way: first, the pituitary in the large toe; then the thyroid; next, the adrenal; and finally, the ankle for the sex glands.

Conditioning the Spleen

Now there are two more important reflexes to stimulate—that for the spleen on the left foot and the one for the liver on the right foot. The spleen is the storage container of our life energy forces and the producer of red blood cells. It is on the left side only, so take your left foot into position and place your fingers just under the little toe. Move down just below this pad and just above the waistline to find this reflex. Work it for about 30 seconds, and while you are in this area, criss-cross the whole pad because you may as well give the heart an extra boost, too, with 15 or 20 seconds of reflex stimulation.

Conditioning the Liver

Do the same for the liver; when reflexing the right foot, cover the space from the waistline up to the diaphragm with a criss-cross technique for 15 or 20 seconds. Work from the outside to the inside of the foot, change hands, and work across in the opposite direction. Reflex the liver to release high-energy glucose, which will help give you a boost of energy.

Final Brushups

Finally, go back and give the reflex to the pituitary on the center of the big toe an extra deep prod or two, as a final signal for it to get busy and help the other glands send you some quick energy.

Complete the regimen by rotating each foot vigorously a few times, using a rolling motion, first to the left and then to the right. (If you are unable to reach your feet, remember to use your Deluxe-Foot-Roller.)

The whole procedure should have taken you less than five minutes; believe me, you will find that you have never spent a more rewarding five minutes, especially when your guests compliment you at the end of an enchanting evening and wonder how you did it all and still managed to look refreshed and full of youthful energy.

REMEMBER YOUR FAMILY AND FRIENDS

Try to keep in mind that other members of the family, or those with whom you work, may be suffering from fatigue without being aware of the reason for their irritability, accompanied by a feeling of futility and depression. There can be no doubt that a constant, nagging sense of fatigue can develop into a person's greatest enemy, depriving him or her of happy, joyful living.

Anxiety, headaches, and nervousness often accompany fatigue. Sleep disorders, complications with sexual function, and lack of concentration are often present as well. It has been known to wreck homes, to shorten life, and it certainly makes life far from enjoyable. It can lead to mental illness. Frequently, fatigue means being more weary on rising than on going to bed and dragging a heavy, overtaxed body around day after day. How pointless it is to allow such a situation to continue when reflexology provides fast, cost-free relief!

Restoring the Energies of a Male Partner

Let's turn our focus to the male partner of the family who may feel unwilling to admit that he is not quite the tower of strength he pretends to be. In his desperate need for sufficient strength to carry through day after day, he may be driven to pep pills or alcoholic drinks which not only provide relief for a very short duration but may also adversely affect his personality. His fatigue may spring from any number of causes. He may snatch a hasty meal which does not contain sufficient nourishment. He may be under constant mental or physical pressure all of which adds to the stress and the drain of energy. At home, he may collapse into a comfortable chair and fall asleep. This is a sign that somewhere the generators of the electric forces are not functioning at full efficiency, that his cells are dying, and that the process of aging is accelerating.

Here is where the knowledgeable partner can take action to restore him to youthful vitality. Make a mild mixture of therapeutic water by adding the juice from 1/2 fresh lemon or lime to 6 ounces of water. If he enjoys scented oils, add five or six drops of plant oil in place of the lemon or lime juice. The scent of eucalyptus or mint is refreshing and energizing for some men.

You (or he) can then bathe his feet with a cool saturated washcloth. Then proceed to give him a quick reflex pickup as outlined in the beginning of this chapter. Watch the change in him and his feelings toward you, as weariness makes room for a new surge of positive energy which floods his entire body as if by a miracle.

In addition to this fast pickup treatment, do a complete reflex workout of both feet to recondition the body just before retiring for the night, or at a time when it can be followed by sleep for an hour or longer.

Restoring Her Energies

Of course, the female partner has an equal need to restore her own depleted energies after a hectic day. She, as well, can become completely overwhelmed with the many demands on her time and strength.

Suggest that she sit down in her favorite chair and take a few deep breaths, slowly inhaling through her nose and exhaling through her mouth. Then help her banish the day's tensions by treating her to a calming reflexology session.

Integrate reflex techniques (found in the first part of this chapter) to relax her, with the same method described earlier for men. However, she may enjoy five or six drops of essential oil in the water rather than the lemon or lime juice. Rosemary and geranium oils are extremely refreshing, and will help to restore her strength and energy, while lavender helps the mind and muscles relax. The combination of the pleasant scent and the stimulation from reflexology will promote internal harmony and create a more cheerful disposition.

Water, lemon, or essential oils can be an added pleasure; however, they are not necessary for total relaxation. You may want to use a washcloth with plain water, or just a couple of baby wipes to clean the feet before working on them.

(Essential oils are condensed fluids that are not oily, and they can be found in your health food store, or wherever aromotherapy products are sold. They come from different herbs and flowers and have a strong effect on the subconscious to relieve mental and physical stress.)

What to Do for Exhausting Shopping Trips

Shopping trips can be real energy robbers. Assume that you and a friend start out fresh and enthusiastic for a day of shopping. You walk the streets, going from store to store, searching for just the right purchase. After hours of walking, there comes a time when you feel ready to collapse on the street, and your enthusiasm is gone. You haven't found what you were looking for after all. Your muscles are protesting and your head is beginning to ache. What can you do for a quick energy pick-up? Take a reflexology tonic as indicated in this chapter.

Find a lounge in one of the stores, or go to your car if you prefer. Take your shoes off and stimulate those pep-restorer reflexes just mentioned.

A Case History of Overcoming Shopping Exhaustion

As proof of the effectiveness of this treatment, let me tell you about a personal experience. With a close friend, I drove about 100 miles to a large city to attend an evening concert. We left early in the morning so that we would have a leisurely day for shopping.

At about one o'clock, my friend began to complain about a headache. She grew more and more tired, and we had to look for a place where she could rest. I offered to reflex her feet if we could find a place where she could sit down. She kept insisting that she would be fine after taking some pills. But before long she felt so exhausted that we went into a lounge in one of the stores, where she collapsed into a chair. I removed her shoes and worked the reflexes to the glands that produce quick energy, and also her big toe to relieve the headache.

While we were doing this, one of the clerks came in. She said, "That looks wonderful to me—I think I'll pull off my shoes and have you rub my feet, too." She seemed to sense instinctively that rubbing the feet is relaxing.

After rubbing my friend's feet, I let her rest quietly for about five minutes. Her headache vanished completely, and she was soon filled with renewed vigor. "It's like getting your second wind," she commented. We finished shopping, had dinner, enjoyed a wonderful concert, and drove 100 miles home late in the evening, all without suffering from the "drag" that often spoils an otherwise pleasant excursion.

QUICK ENERGY ENHANCEMENT FOR TRAVEL EXHAUSTION

You may be a professional athlete who travels with a team, a truck driver, or traveling salesperson, or you may be one of those unfortunate people who cannot take very much traveling without feeling drained of all energy after a few hours of driving or riding. Or perhaps you are a senior citizen who would like to take one of those interesting bus excursions but do not feel that you have the energy to travel that far.

Even if there is no one available who can give you a mini reflex workout, you can help yourself to renewed energy and a feeling of well-being by studying the charts and applying the simple techniques of foot reflexology. And this can be done without resorting to drugs or other artificial pep-boosters which leave you in the same weary condition, if not worse, when their effects wear off.

Reflexology Tips When Traveling with the Family

The average vacationing family tries to cover too many miles in a hurry, which results with the children getting restless and tired. Traveling with a family means many hectic demands on mind and body, not only for the driver but for everyone else in the vehicle. It is no wonder that so many people simply say, "It isn't worth it!" But if everyone in the family learns the way to give a fast pick-up by stimulating the reflexes of the feet, any vacation can be a pleasant experience.

When the children become irritable and restless, have them give each other a foot workout which will quiet them down. In the evening, take turns reflexing each other's feet, and you will enjoy a good night's rest and wake ready for another memorable day.

But let me give you a word of caution: *Don't forget that reflexology can be very relaxing even if given for only a few seconds.* This is fine for the children for they will fall asleep, or at least be less quarrelsome. But if the treatment lasts more than five minutes, be sure that you can lie down and sleep for an hour or so before trying to drive again.

Although a quick energy pick-up workout can be given any time weariness begins to set in, the best time for a good overall treatment is just before going to bed. You will be so relaxed that you will sleep like a baby, as the saying goes. You will also awaken with all the bounce and energy of youth, and be able to look forward with great anticipation and eagerness to another travel day.

Reflexology for Campers

A pick-up tonic through foot reflexology is exactly what every amateur outdoor sportsman, hunter, or fisherman is looking for after a hard day's exertion. Your first move in getting back to camp is to get out of your wet clothes immediately. If a meal is ready for you, sit down and eat. If not, and you are too tired to fix something, turn to the feet for a fast camper's pick-up tonic!

It is better to have someone else give you a reflex workout, one who understands the technique of reflexology. But if necessary, give yourself a treatment.

Take off your shoes and socks, and start working the feet as described. If you are very cold and your feet are wet, just rub them briskly for a few minutes before starting to work the reflexes. You will be surprised to see how quickly this warms you all over, and after digging and prodding and massaging the reflexes in both feet, you will feel a warm glow spreading over your entire body.

If you do not intend to go to bed right away, however, do not reflex the entire foot as you will become very sleepy. For just a quick energy pick-up, remember to work the big toe and under it (pituitary and thyroid), then the center section of the bottom of both feet (for the adrenal glands), under the ankle bones (for the gonads), and on the left foot across the ball of the foot and under the little toe pad for the spleen and the heart, and a short reflex to the same area on the right foot—to stimulate the liver. Incidentally, this reflex routine is good to use whenever you are out exerting yourself in ways your body is not accustomed to, in order to give it an extra boost of energy.

What Every Part-time Sports Enthusiast Must Know About Heart Attacks

Opening day of skiing, fishing, baseball, or any other sporting season often brings countless reports of sudden heart attacks suffered by sports enthusiasts of all ages. Long periods of inactivity have left the heart unprepared for the sudden surge of adrenaline which is rushed to this blood-pumping organ at the first sign of excitement. Remember that the heart is really a large muscle, and that an easy life keeps it pumping slowly. Thus it becomes soft from lack of exercise, just like any other muscle which has become weakened under routine activities. When the adrenal gland is stimulated by excitement, the heart speeds up its rhythm and pumps at a much faster rate. Sometimes it cannot take such a sudden change of pace without causing great discomfort or even a heart attack.

If a heart attack should occur when the victim is miles away from a doctor, first work the reflexes across the chest area, top and bottom of left foot. Then continue to work under and all over the little toe. Move to the reflex of the pituitary in the center of the big toe for a few seconds of reflex stimulation, and return to the little toe area. Again reflex across the whole chest area, using the criss-cross technique, working top and sole of foot.

It is, in fact, a good idea to give yourself a reflex workout any time that you feel odd in any way while out hiking or participating in a sports event that you have not been active in for awhile. Just sit down, take off your shoes, and rub the reflex area between the waistline and diaphragm, also around your little toe and under it for a few minutes. Dig in deeply, even if you have to use a stick. If you can't reach your feet, and there is a rocky area nearby, walk over it in your bare feet. Of course, it will hurt! But that is better than having a disabling illness strike you, isn't it? It may forestall an impending heart attack, and in any event, it will recharge your vitality and give you strength either to get to a doctor or to go on with the hike or activity, if you are merely fatigued.

REFLEXOLOGY FOR LEG CRAMPS

Leg cramps in muscles unused to sudden demands are a common complaint of outdoorsmen and athletes. Familiarity with reflexology is the answer to get fast relief.

A few years ago a friend and I took our places near a certain path early one morning, to wait for a large buck which, we were told, came down the mountain every day just about dawn. We sat motionlessly, watching the trail. Just when it was time for the deer to show, my friend whispered, "I have a terrible cramp in my leg. I'm sorry, but I've just got to move." Both of us realized that to make a move at that crucial moment would give our presence away. I reached over quietly and massaged the cords in back of his knee for a few minutes and told him to point his toe up toward his nose. This relaxed the cramped muscles in his leg, and he was able to sit patiently until the unsuspecting deer appeared. Without knowledge of reflexology, we would have missed seeing one of the most beautiful animals on this planet.

HOT WEATHER FATIGUE

Does hot weather leave you depleted of energy? Foot reflexology is the answer. If you are not one of those fortunate people who can boast of "thriving" on hot weather, chances are you suffer from the weary feeling known as "heat exhaustion."

When a hot day drains you of energy, just find a nice, shady nook, bare your feet if they are not already bare, and give them a workout that will stimulate the glands that recharge the entire body.

Work the reflex to the pituitary gland in the center of the big toe to stimulate it into action so that it can start sending energy to the thyroid, adrenals, spleen, and gonads. Once you get them into action, they will stimulate the rest of the body.

In this chapter, you have been given the "recipe" for a fast pick-up tonic to use whenever you feel low in vitality. Apply this reflex workout to the same glands for hot weather fatigue, and you will feel refreshed and invigorated as if by magic.

HOW TO DISSOLVE STRESS WITH REFLEXOLOGY

Various studies show that many health problems are instigated by emotions. This is referred to as the "mind-body connection." People who live in constant tension often find that they are more likely to be contenders for such ailments as high blood pressure, headaches, back pain, ulcers, mental disorders, and even rheumatoid arthritis, more so than those who do not experience prolonged stress or anxiety.

Emotional stress usually implies a conflict of circumstances for which there seems to be no appropriate solution. Professional life is often highly competitive and places us under heavy pressures which are often responsible for much pain and suffering. This type of stress cannot be completely avoided; however, it can be minimized.

If you find yourself in a challenging situation such as when you know the important decision you make will affect other people and you are not sure whether to follow your heart or your intellect, remember you have the power within to balance your emotions and wisdom so that the decisions you make will be right for everyone involved.

There are various methods you can learn for facing emotional challenges that will enable you to carry responsibility without excessive stress. Try these three steps.

Three Easy Steps to Stop Stress

The first step is to find an ideal location, one where you can relax. Then kick off your shoes and slowly and gently work the reflexes to the pituitary, work all the endocrine reflexes, the spine reflex, over the tops and on the bottoms of your feet, one foot at a time. Slowly work up the back of the leg and around the ankles, too. This workout should take about five minutes on each foot.

The second step is to sit back, elevate your feet, and clear your mind. Close your eyes and visualize your stress as a frozen pond. The pond is cold and hard and nothing can get through it. Nothing, that is, except nature. Now here comes the sunshine, and little by little the ice starts to melt (just like your stress, little by little, leaving your body). Soon the warm sun melts all the ice and, drop by drop, the water in the little pond becomes soft and warm again. (Just as you relax, one by one all the tensions melt away, leaving you completely relaxed, both emotionally and physically.) If time permits, take a short nap.

The third step is to take several slow, deep breaths and do some stretching exercises to loosen up. Work over the tops and sides of your feet with quick movements for one or two minutes, just enough to get your circulation moving. Now drink a glass of cool water and you are ready to go. Your thoughts will be clear and reliable, your attitude considerate and good-natured. You will no longer feel the drain of stress; instead you will have renewed strength, prepared to accomplish anything.

Restore Your Body's Chemical Balance

When the body experiences stress for a prolonged period of time, it responds with high blood pressure, an increased heartbeat, muscles that contract, or a stomach that produces additional digestive juices. Even the adrenals may start pumping out too much adrenaline, and before you know it, the body chemistry level is disturbed.

To be healthy, the body needs the right chemical balance—just as plants need the right amount of soil and water to produce beautiful flowers; just as car engines need the correct amount of oil and gas to run efficiently.

Although many things contribute to stress, you can stop unwanted stress-related illnesses. Simply take the time to care about your health. Get in touch with nature, and use reflexology as a safe and natural way to restore health and harmony to your body. You will notice dramatic changes as you relax totally. Your muscles will unwind, your heartbeat will slow down; soon you'll feel more at ease, thereby fending off disease.

Use Slow, Tranquil Pressure

Find an ideal location, one where you can relax. Remove your shoes and gently use your thumb to work the reflexes of the endocrine glands. These glands are mostly lined up in the center core of your body; therefore, their reflex areas are mostly lined up along the inner side of each foot. All, that is, except the protected sex gland reflexes, which are under the ankles. (Refer to Chart E, page 12.)

Remember the pituitary gland is in your brain; when you are agitated, or worked up, this master gland tells the other glands to react in the same way. The adrenal gland reacts to intense emotions via the sympathetic nervous system. When you are stressed, tense, frightened, or angry, this gland produces hormones that cause the blood pressure to rise, muscles to tighten, and pupils to widen.

To sedate the chemical substances (hormones) going into your bloodstream, you will want to work the pituitary and adrenal gland reflexes with slow, tranquil pressure. This will send the "signal" to calm down. Reflexing in this manner encourages the glands to produce hormones that balance the body and make it feel at ease.

Additional reflex areas to help relax stress and tensions are the spine reflex, as well as those over the tops of both feet, up the back of each leg and all around the ankles.

This workout should take about five minutes on each foot.

Use Deluxe-Foot-Roller to Reduce Stress

The Deluxe-Foot-Roller is a reflexology self-help tool (see Photo 3 on page 34) that relaxes built-up frustrations and dissolves stress. It is easy to use at home, at work, or on vacation. Just sit on the sofa or in a comfortable chair; place the roller on the floor in front of you, put one foot on its center, very *slowly* push your foot forward and then pull it backward. The roller will move easily as the small nodules press into the reflexes on the bottom of your feet to stimulate renewed circulation throughout your whole body.

The roller has higher nodules on one side, which conform well to the instep of the foot. As you move your foot over the roller, the larger side reaches into the spinal column reflex area, as well as into the endocrine reflexes for a more thorough workout. Or use both feet on the round disks at the ends of your roller to calm the mind and relax the body. Use the technique most comfortable for you. Your aim is to decrease tension and tone the body. As you reduce stress you bring healthy changes to all systems.

To accelerate the relaxing process, breathe from your diaphragm rather than from your chest. Remember, when tension blocks the natural flow, congestion and disease can occur. Don't let this happen to you.

When tensions are reduced and your body becomes totally relaxed, you will notice a dramatic change in the way you feel. Breathing and heartbeat will return to normal and internal systems and muscles will ease up, thus causing blood and lymph circulation to improve. This is a healthful method of relieving stress and tensions, and promotes deep relaxation, the key to effective healing.

CHAPTER 27

How to Have More "Go Power" with Reflexology

I have told you how to relax and how to overcome various illnesses. Now I would like to tell you how to use reflexology as your "go power," how to recharge your vitality and give yourself a pick-up that will last all day.

HOW TO GET STARTED FOR THE DAY

One of my patients told me that she had a hard time getting up in the morning. "It just seemed that I couldn't get awake, or make my body respond without a great effort," she said. "Then I would wander around in a daze for an hour or more before I could get in gear and move and think normally. One morning I had a lot of work ahead of me. As I opened my eyes I thought of all the work I had to get done that day, and I wished that I could feel full of pep and vitality and be able to jump out of bed and pitch into it, instead of dragging around for an hour drinking coffee for a stimulant.

"As I lay there I thought of reflexology. If it worked to relax you when you were tired, why couldn't it pep you up when you needed a stimulant in the morning?" She went on to tell me that she curled around in bed and started to reflex her feet as I had shown her. "I decided if the pituitary reflex relaxed, then it should also be able to

204

give some 'go power,' so I gave both big toes a good working over. Then I worked my thumb on down under the big toe bone where you had shown me the reflex to the thyroid was located and gave that a couple of pushes. If anyone ever needed a push button to start one's motor going with a zing, I needed it this particular morning, so I covered my feet quickly with the rolling push-and-pull motion that you had taught me. I don't think the whole procedure took me over two minutes, but by the time I was finished, I felt wide awake. I got out of bed and was so full of energy I started in on my work before I realized that I had not had my coffee yet. No more lying in bed dreading to get up for me," she said. "I felt wonderful the rest of the day."

Working these reflexes in the bottom of your feet is like opening up a new power within you. Nearly everyone today knows that we are filled with a great power likened to TNT—yes, even the atomic bomb, which is merely atoms exploding for the will of man.

Our bodies are as subject to the rhythmic laws of nature and the universe as the planet is in its revolution around the sun.

Everything is in a state of vibration. There is nothing in absolute rest; from the greatest sun to the tiniest atom, there is motion and vibration. Do you know that if atoms were deprived of vibration, it is said, it would wreck the universe? Matter is constantly played upon by energy and countless forms result, and yet even the forms are not permanent; they begin to change the moment they are created and from them are born new forms, which in turn change and give rise to newer forms, and so on.

In like manner, the atoms in the human body are in constant vibration. Changes are occurring unceasingly. There is almost a complete change in the matter composing the body within a few months. Nothing is permanent in the world of forms; they are but appearances and they come and they go—constant vibration—constant change.

REFLEXOLOGY, THE NATURAL PRIMER

So in reflexology we have the natural method of sending these powerful vibrations to any spot in our body, thus recharging the atoms with a shot of power through the reflexes. We might say we are transferring the power within our bodies to places where we need a burst of energy for a quick pick-up, or to stimulate the atoms in a certain sluggish area to a new surge of circulation, life, and energy. If the matter of our bodies is in constant change at a certain rate of vibration, and if in all vibration there is found to be a certain rhythm, then you can see how simple it is for Nature to heal any and all disturbances in the body if given a chance to vibrate in rhythm.

Our bodies are as subject to rhythmic laws as is the planet in its revolution around the sun. So we turn to reflexology and work the reflexes in the bottoms of the feet to get the body back into its natural rhythm with the universe.

If a high note is sounded repeatedly and in rhythm, it will start into motion vibrations that can bring down a building. Picture soldiers marching in rhythm across a bridge; their vibrations could bring the bridge down. These manifestations of the effect rhythmic motion has on matter will give you an idea of how important rhythm and harmony are to the health of our bodies.

This is why so many people seemingly have every gland and organ in their bodies malfunctioning in one way or another. How can a body run smoothly and in perfect health if the instruments are out of tune, such as the glands and the organs? Any one of them can start a chain reaction of disharmony and illness. So many people come to me with the same story, "I don't know what is the matter with me. I am just sick all over. The doctors don't know either; they say it is my mind. But I can't eat; if I do, it makes me sick. I am losing weight and I have no energy, as I used to."

Why the Whole Body Must Be Stimulated With Reflexology

These people cannot be helped by treating just one part of the body. The whole body has become out of tune and the vibrations of its atoms are not changing in a perfect pattern of health, because somewhere some gland has been allowed to get out of harmony. To restore perfect health, we will have to get our vibrations back into rhythm and our glands and organs back into tune with each other so that they can send harmonious vibrations into every atom that is busy trying to build the body back to the full strength of every cell.

This is why reflexology brings about such seeming miracles. Actually it is a very simple and natural process of tuning the instruments of the body: just press the reflexes in the bottoms of the feet to break up the congestion that has slowed down the circulation of the life forces to certain glands and organs. All body cells will be energized by the radiations of vital force when the reflexes are used to awaken these glands to their natural functions.

By working the reflex to the pituitary you are tuning the main gland, as you would tune the leading violin in a symphony orchestra. This gland, which has its reflex in the center of the big toe, is the pep gland. It also has a direct bearing on the sex glands which are responsible for our personalities and our drive, our get-up-and-go, our vitality and energy.

This is the way our bodies harmonize with the symphony of the universe when they are in perfect tune. But can you imagine how an orchestra would sound if just one instrument were out of tune? You can see how impossible it is for us to have good health and energy if some part of our body malfunctions.

Reflexology is the only method I know of that works on the whole body at the same time, leaving no instrument or gland untouched, as the feet are completely covered by stimulation. There is no part left out unless you miss it as you reflex the entire left and right feet.

HOW REFLEXOLOGY REVITALIZES ALL OF YOU

It seems that men or women who are very successful will be the ones with a strong sex drive, and the endocrine glands have to be in good health for them to have this sex drive. If you are not mentally alert and don't want to work for success, then you probably lack a strong sex drive and will be content to sit and let the world go by, unless you stimulate the endocrine glands to normal action. And the most natural and simplest way to do this is by working the reflexes to all of these glands.

We have discussed both the pituitary gland and the hypothalamus and their reflexes in the big toe. The next gland is also in the head and is stimulated in the big toe also; only instead of working in the center, we move the finger over to the side toward the second toe to find the reflex to the pineal gland. If the reflex to the pituitary is tender, then this will also probably be quite sensitive when pressed on. Then we go to the reflexes to the thyroid gland just under the bone of the big toe, and the parathyroids in the same location as the thyroid. However, the parathyroids are deeper and more pressure must be put into their reflexing if they need special attention; otherwise they will receive enough stimulation as you work the thyroid reflex.

The thymus is important, too, and has a reflex in each foot almost up at the root of the big toes.

Then we go to the adrenals, whose reflexes are in the center of each foot. And remember, they, like the sex glands, give you "go power," drive to act, untiring energy.

Next is the pancreas gland, larger than the other endocrine glands, which lies behind the lower part of the stomach. This is the gland that produces insulin, among other things. Anyone suffering from diabetes is familiar with the feeling of weakness suffered when this gland is not working properly and fails to supply a sufficient amount of insulin.

So we would work the reflexes to this all-important gland along the waistline of each foot. Since this reflex is close to that of the stomach, it will get the benefit of the stimulation when you work the stomach reflex. And in doing this particular work you also help digestion in two ways because the pancreas is also a producer of pancreatic juice containing enzymes important in digestion.

We then work the reflexes to the gonads (sex glands) which are, as you will remember, in the area of the ankles. It is well to reflex all around the ankles on the inside and outside of both feet, and up the back of the leg just above the heel on both sides of the cord extending up the back of the leg, as this whole area has reflexes to the reproductive glands.

By massaging the whole foot, all the cells are stimulated because the circulation is released to allow the natural life force to bring renewed vigor to every part of the body. In this way the vibrations of the life force restore harmony and health to every part of the body.

The little gland called the spleen is not only a builder of red blood cells to keep you full of health and pep, but it is also a storehouse of the life force that we receive from the surrounding air. Many medical centers are starting to understand this life force, which is called "prana" by the yogis. It is truly an electrical life force and without it nothing can live.

So keep your spleen healthy by working the reflex to it which is located under the pad on your left foot. See Chart B for exact location to reflex. When one uses a Deluxe-Foot-Roller, the whole foot tingles with healing vibrations and the reflexes are easily reached without bending over. Roll it quickly beneath each foot so that it thoroughly and easily reaches all reflex buttons to give you a blast of renewed energy.

When this life force is distributed over the entire body through the etheric networks, it radiates an aura of health. If you want your aura to reflect perfect health and energy and your body to vibrate in tune with the symphony of the universe, keep it in perfect condition by stimulating the reflexes in the bottoms of your feet as indicated in this book.

Part Three

How You Can Help Others with Reflexology

Reflexology Tips and Techniques for Helping Others

You have just been given the information needed to help yourself take an active part in the care of your own health with foot reflexology. Now you have the opportunity to learn how, by this natural science of healing, you can help your family and friends. With the knowledge and skills you acquire from this book, you will have the potential, not only to protect your own health, but to help people everywhere enhance their health and the quality of their lives.

Health is something that you cannot afford to take chances with. Recognizing the symptoms and reflexes that "signal" emotional or physical illness is the first step to preventing disease. Continue the healing steps by working sore reflex areas. Your aim is to relieve tensions and promote circulation to unblock vital energies. When the body regains its internal strength, it has the ability to heal itself and to bring prompt and effective relief from many types of ailments.

In this section we will not go into detailed study of diseases, circulation or the nervous system, but will concentrate on where the reflexes are located, and how they can be stimulated to renew the circulation of vital energy to restore the body to normal health.

We suggest that you read the first and second parts of this book completely so that you will become familiar with the amazing results of reflexology. This will also instruct you about the importance of the body's various systems, and how they are all interrelated. After discovering the benefits on yourself, you will be ready to learn the proper reflex techniques to help others improve, maintain, and preserve good health.

PREPARATIONS FOR GIVING REFLEXOLOGY

It may take some time before you are able to memorize pressure points. Look at the foot reflexology chart (Chart B in Chapter 2). Or you can purchase a large wall-size chart and post it on the wall behind the person you are working on. This way you will be facing the chart, and can refer to it easily while doing your reflex work. (See back of book, for ordering information.) To be fully successful, be sensitive to the needs and to the level of tolerance of your partner. Use the appropriate pressure, never gouge, and be careful not to let your finger or thumbnails poke or injure the feet you work on.

Giving reflexology is special, and only a comprehensive knowledge of this field will give you that necessary air of confidence and skill required to improve another person's life.

For Best Results Create a Comfortable Environment

Relaxation is the key to effective reflexology. Before you start your reflex work, make sure the room is comfortably warm and calm. There should be a pleasant setting and a minimum of noise. Soft music of the reflex receiver's choice may create a pleasant and relaxing atmosphere; others, however, find that music of any kind interferes with relaxation.

If the receiver's feet feel cold to your hands, you may want to leave a sock on one foot. If at home, put a slipper on or cover one foot with a blanket while you are working the other. Remember that feet are usually within warm shoes and socks, and can become quite cold when exposed to the open air. Lights should be soft, so as not to interfere with the complete relaxation of your partner's eyes. If, at all possible, try to maintain privacy during the reflex session.

How to Provide Comfort and a Sense of Well-being

Reflexology can be given almost anywhere, and at any time, but when possible, you should provide a relaxed, comfortable setting to be most effective. The most comfortable and relaxing position for both you and your reflex partner will be the most beneficial. The person receiving reflexology should sit in a chair that has a high back, one that gives firm support to the head and back. It should be large and sturdy enough to accommodate body size to allow complete relaxation.

A reclining chair, with attached foot rest, offers the ideal position. The foot lift should come up high enough for you to be able to sit comfortably in an ordinary chair in front of your reflex partner, so you can reach the feet without strain. If your partner is in a recliner, make sure that you lower the back rest of the chair slowly, as a sudden leaning back may be frightening. Always be gentle and considerate, whether you are working on your grandmother or the well-muscled athlete of the family, because there may be apprehension or fear of being hurt when you first start reflexing.

An ill person may be particularly sensitive, feel unsure, or be extremely fatigued. Always be kind and understanding in bringing relief in the quickest and most natural way possible, through reflexology.

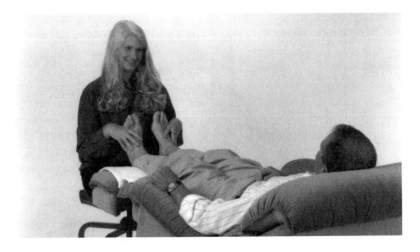

Photo 28. Choose a position that is comfortable for both the person giving, and the one receiving reflexology. Place your thumbs on the soles of your partner's feet, while your fingers wrap around the sides and over the top. Use a press-and-slide movement from the heels upward past the toes. (Work one or two feet at a time.) Repeat several times to relax muscle and nerve tension. This is a nice technique to use at the beginning of each session.

If you are outside working, camping, hiking, or at a sports event with no comfortable chair available, have the person sit on the floor (or ground) and lean up against the wall (or a tree) for back support. Always make sure the area is safe, and comfortable, for positive results. You can then sit comfortably in front of them and apply reflexology to one foot at a time. After all, if someone you are with is stressed, tired, or has a related illness and needs your assistance as a reflexologist, how can you refuse?

When giving reflexology to a person in bed, you can sit on the bed, in a chair beside it, or you can work from the end of the bed.

Using the Correct Pressure

It has been scientifically established that when reflexology is given for invigorating purposes, the pressure should be deep and the hands should move quickly. This will stimulate the blood circulation and help the receiver feel alert and full of vitality. When soothing or relaxing benefits are sought, however, you will want to use a light touch, with slow, smooth, and even pressure.

Reflexology requires strong hands, and your fingers may become tired and sore if you work on more than one person a day. You may use your knuckles on some reflex areas, or place one thumb on top of another for added strength.

The Reflex Probe can be very helpful in your reflex work (see Photo 25, page 157). Some reflexes are located so deep that you just cannot reach them without a tool of some kind, especially on most men because of the thicker and tougher covering on the soles. However, it is not advisable to use the Reflex Probe until you have mastered the use of your thumb. With time and practice you will become more familiar with the amount of pressure that is needed to accomplish good results without bruising the skin or the tiny capillaries close to the surface.

Always be careful not to create any black-and-blue bruise spots on anyone's feet. This "feel" for the right pressure will come to you with practice. If bruises do appear, the blood which has collected under the skin, causing the discoloration, is usually absorbed gradually without any discomfort. To hasten this process, hold your reflexpartner's foot in both hands and rub it gently. You might wait a few days before continuing with reflexology on this person, especially on the discolored parts of the feet.

What to Do If Reflexology Is Painful

If your partner finds the first reflex session painful, explain that the pain is the "clue" to any ailments, and that the tenderness will disappear as accumulated congestion and poisons in the body are dissipated by the reflex work. Ask your partner to tell you about any sharp pain, and use the gentlest possible pressure on that reflex "button." There is no point in hurting the feet more than necessary.

Go on working the other reflexes, returning to the painful one from time to time, and you will find the tenderness disappearing little by little with each touch as the reflex sends its healing forces surging back to the ailing organ it represents.

Maintaining a Positive Attitude Is Beneficial to Healing

When someone you love and care about is suffering from an illness, your kind and loving attitude when you are doing your reflex work will be beneficial. Reemphasize that you will stop at any time if so requested.

If the idea of reflexology is initially uncomfortable, start out by just holding one foot at a time within your healing hands to help your partner feel relaxed. In this way you can relieve distress, worry, and fear. Use warm genuine expressions and share kind positive thoughts about the natural benefits of reflexology. Quote some case histories from the first and second parts of this book, or from one of our other books, where the healing energies of reflexology has helped others.

Once your reflex companion is comfortable with the idea of using reflex stimulation to balance the various systems of the body, you can proceed with the reflexology session. Continue with loving words, compassion, and understanding. When you are completely open to feelings and needs, you can respond in a way that will encourage and uplift your partner. It is very important to exude confidence about the return of good health. And as you notice this occurring, encourage a renewed interest in life, in hobbies. Take a walk with them, and work to rebuild a reinvigorated spirit. You will be amazed at the quick recovery, as nature does the healing!

A Personal Touch

There is a difference between giving oneself a reflex workout, and reflexing another person who may be seeking relief from pain, stress, or illness.

As you learn how to give reflexology, you may want to find a reflex partner to study with you. This way you can practice on each other. However, since reflexology must be limited to a few minutes per session at intervals of every other day for the first week, it is not advisable to practice on only one person. Give different members of your family a practice workout, until you discover where the reflexes are hidden under the skin and inside the foot.

Preparing to Give Reflexology

When preparing to give reflexology to a friend whose feet you have "not met" before, you should always ask if there have ever been any foot troubles, such as broken bones from accidents, corrective surgery on toes, or other such complications. Also check the feet for bunions, corns, or toenail troubles. You need to be gentle in these areas.

If the feet perspire excessively, use a baby wipe to clean them gently, then dust them lightly with cornstarch. Baby powder is not good, as it tends to become airborne and the fine powder could be inhaled into the lungs. On hot days it is very natural for feet to perspire.

Feet are a wondrous masterpiece of anatomical engineering and should not be taken for granted. Health is vital to a person's whole well-being; when your feet hurt, you hurt all over.

How to Find Reflex Locations on Another Person's Feet

When you use the practical and immediately available techniques of reflexology on yourself, it helps you identify with the guidelines of the feet, as well as experience various pressures and techniques. As you develop a feeling for this healing energy, you will want to share it with others. To prepare yourself for all the different types of feet (thin and

BONES OF THE FOOT

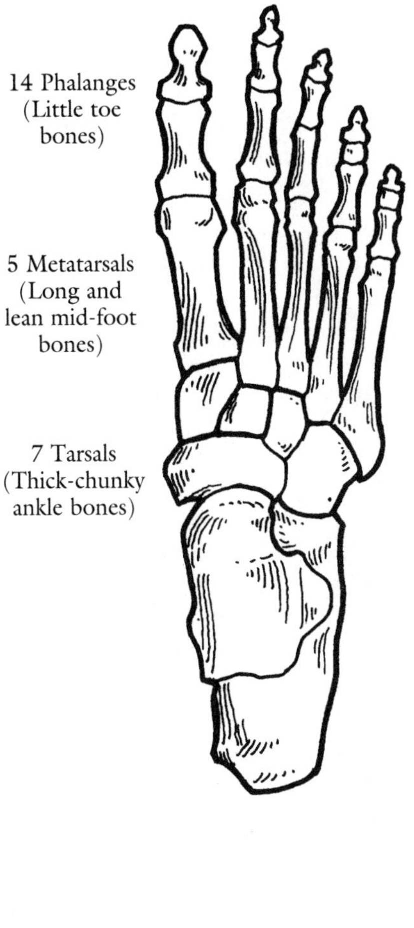

BASIC REFLEX INDENTIFICATION AREAS

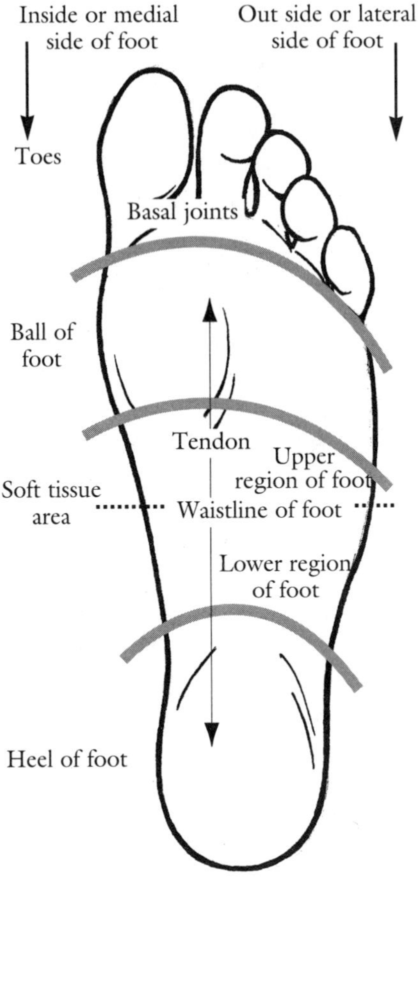

14 Phalanges
(Little toe
bones)

5 Metatarsals
(Long and
lean mid-foot
bones)

7 Tarsals
(Thick-chunky
ankle bones)

Inside or medial
side of foot

Out side or lateral
side of foot

Toes

Basal joints

Ball of
foot

Tendon

Upper
region of foot

Soft tissue
area

Waistline of foot

Lower region
of foot

Heel of foot

CHART I. The bone structure of the foot is divided into three groups and consists of 26 bones. Study the internal bone structure and external regions of the foot. This will be helpful when you are searching for tender reflex areas under the skin.

boney, high and low arches, short and wide, etc.) look at Chart I for the basic bone structure and external regions of the foot. This will assist you in finding the exact location of each reflex area. Also refer to Charts B, C, and D as needed.

LEARN THE BASIC TECHNIQUES TO HELP OTHERS

Learning different techniques is fun and easy, and will enhance your reflex sessions more effectively. Proper knowledge of how to use both hands in a "team" effort will improve your skills as a good reflexologist. (See Chapter 5.) Studying these techniques will insure greater accuracy and smoothness.

When giving reflexology to someone else, remember the importance of showing that you truly care about your partner's health and well-being. As you develop reflex sensitivity, you will be able to add your own personal touch to the reflex sessions. Along with special care and sincere dedication, your techniques will help to soothe away stress and help your reflex companion regain strength and vitality.

Starting the Reflex Session

You now have your partner resting comfortably, with the soles of the feet facing you. Make necessary observations of the feet for current or past injuries; check for bruises and callouses and avoid working on these sensitive areas at this time. Since the initial contact with another person's feet is important, we like to start the reflexology techniques with a soft gentle touch. First give a tender "hello hug" to the top of both feet. Then with both hands give each foot a gentle squeeze. Hug the tops, bottoms and sides of each foot. (See Illustration 7c on page 51; and photo 28 on page 215.)

If your partner seems to be suffering from mental or physical stress, you will want to create an atmosphere of tranquility. So start the reflex session with one or two relaxation techniques to help relax the feet and body.

Wringing the Foot

You have just given each foot a "hello hug"; now, while you have the foot in this position, you can also release negative tensions with a simple method of wringing the foot.

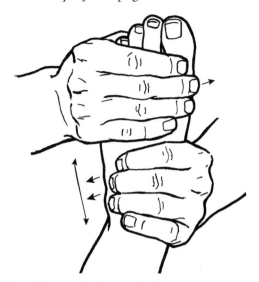

Illustration 18.   Wring each foot to loosen nerves.

To do this you simply place both hands around the foot, fingers facing opposite directions, as though you were going to wring water from a wet towel. Gently push each hand forward (each hand will move in a different direction), tenderly and smoothly wring from the toes, move toward the middle, and gently wring the foot; then move to the ankle area and wring the foot. Switch hands and carefully wring the foot again in the opposite direction. Gradually return to the toes. Repeat on the other foot.

"Press-and-Slide" Thumbs and Fingers to Relax Nerves

Reflexology is most effective when the body is at ease and totally relaxed. If your partner seems stressed, you will want to start the session with one or two routines relaxing to the body and nerves. Start out with the "press-and-slide" technique. Simply rest the feet on a pillow, foot stool, or in your lap, and gently alternate both hands, working one foot at a time.

A. To do this, place both thumbs on the heel of one foot (fingers will be on top of foot); now slide each thumb from the center of the sole to the edges of the foot; alternate your thumbs by using the right and then left thumb as you work up the foot toward the toes.

B. Now repeat the procedure concentrating on top of each foot by alternating your fingers from the center of the foot to the outside edge. Use an upward sweeping motion and work from just above the ankle to the toes. Use relaxing movements; do not appear to be in a hurry or to be rushed in any way. Remember, of course, to do both feet. (See Illustrations 7a and 7b on page 51.)

The Ankle Shuttle and the Metatarsal Squeeze

Do you realize that the average feet will travel over 100,000 miles in a lifetime, even more if their owner is into exercise and running? This is true, so please take good care of these very precious vehicles and give them some special attention whenever possible.

Here are three special methods of relaxing the feet leisurely (as well as calming the whole body luxuriously). Use these techniques after you have reflexed a painful section of the foot, or use them as a method of making very tired feet just plain "feel-great"!

A. Start by placing the fingers upward, keeping inner sides of both hands against either side of the foot. Place a slight pressure toward each hand, then gently roll the foot back and forth between the hands. Start where the toes join the foot, and move toward ankles.

B. The Ankle Shuttle is a little different: point all fingers toward your reflex companion; open hands until your little fingers are beneath the ankles. Now, with the foot between the edges of your hands, gently push and pull your hands in a sawing motion. (Do not lose contact

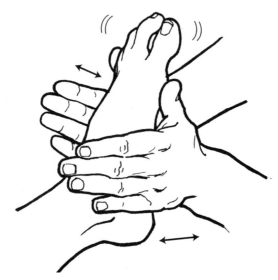

Illustration 19a.   Use the Foot Shuttle to relax the whole body.

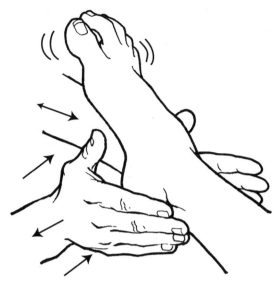

Illustration 19b. Shuttle the foot just below the ankle.

with foot, as this could cause skin irritation.) The foot will rock from side to side; this brings about a soothing as well as a stimulating effect.

C. To alleviate stress from the foot, try this simple method of spreading the left foot out. Place one hand on top of foot, and press down; make a fist with the other hand and press against the sole of

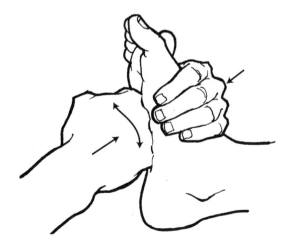

Illustration 19c. The Metatarsal Squeeze feels good, helps to soothe the feet, and is very calming.

the foot. Push in firmly, but gently, with the fist and twist a little to the left and then to the right, while reinforcing the top of the foot with the opposite hand. Now stop pressing with the fist, and squeeze slightly with the hand on top. Repeat this several times, working from the toes to the heel, then back to the toes. This is very soothing and calming to the receiver.

Solar-Plexus-Press

This technique can be used at the beginning *and* at the end of your reflex routine to calm anxiety, release up-tight nerves, and banish tensions. It is important to release all stress, as tautness in the nerves can cause high blood pressure. This slow, calming technique, which brings a sense of peace and harmony to the session, also sends currents of healing energy to both adrenal glands, calming the flow of blood, thereby helping to reduce high blood pressure.

With both feet facing you, your companion should rest them on your lap, a foot stool, or bed. This gives your hands freedom to press your thumbs into both solar plexus points at the same time. Using your two hands, wrap fingers around both of your partner's feet, and place one thumb into the reflex of the solar plexus in the center of each foot. Press with a slow smooth motion. Ask your partner to breathe deeply (you can breathe along as well) and to close his or her eyes for additional relaxation. As you release the pressure, also release your breath, and coach your partner to do the same. Repeat two or three times. All relaxation techniques should be done in a slow rhythmic manner. See Photo 38 on page 305.

Give Nature Time to Repair and Restore the Body to Good Health

At times you may need to become a "reflex-detective" to find out what is causing a certain ailment. You will search the feet for clues (which will show up as sore spots). Tenderness will be a sign that there is congestion or damage within the corresponding part of the body. Your assignments as a reflex-detective are first to read this book, study the charts, and learn where the pressure points are. Then, using the correct method, you will take your time and gently work the sensitivity out of the painful reflex areas.

As a good undercover agent you will use evidence found in the sore reflexes as a key to unlock the mystery causing your friend's discomfort or illness. Application to these tender reflex areas will send a healing energy that corresponds to the organ, gland, or part of the body which is affected. As the vital life forces start surging through the body, the living tissues within the neural pathways will become electrically charged and activate the body's own healing powers.

You will remember to give nature the time needed to repair and restore the body to renewed health. It takes time and perseverance to regain good health, often several days, weeks, months or maybe even years. After all, very little is overcome in the twinkling of an eye. However, with reflexology, I have seen it happen.

BEGINNING THE REFLEX WORKOUT

It is important to first reflex the big toes, as they correspond to the brain. (Often professional reflexologists will work all the toes first, to stimulate energy to the brain. Then they will proceed by working all the other reflex points, which correspond to the core of the body.) However, you are interested simply in learning how to help your family and friends, so begin the reflex session by working one entire foot (toes first, of course), then change feet, and work the other entire foot.

It is important to reflex the big toe first to stimulate renewed circulation to the brain. Neurons in the brain control the body's involuntary activities, such as breathing, digestion, heartbeat, and circulation. It is your aim to stimulate renewed circulation throughout the body, and where better to start than with the brain?

The brain gets its energy from blood that is filled with oxygen and glucose. As the reflexes in the big toe are pressed, various neurological pathways are opened up and circulation of the blood is improved, thus helping to energize the brain cells. With renewed energy, the brain will have better control of the fundamental activities in the body.

Working the Left Foot First

Let's start with the left foot, because it is important that circulation be motivated on the left side of the body first. The reason is that it is from the left side of the body that the heart pumps out oxygen-rich blood, which then travels up to the head and down to the internal organs, as well as to both arms and legs. (The right side of the body returns oxygen-poor blood back to the heart.)

It is, of course, important to stimulate both sides of the body and both feet should be equally reflexed. However, by using reflexology on the left side first, you open up the energy pathways that will encourage the needed oxygenated and nutrient-laden blood to circulate throughout the body.

Work One Foot at a Time

When giving a complete reflex workout you will work the left foot first, for the reason we have explained earlier. Do not change feet until you have mastered every reflex in this foot. (This does not apply when you are giving a mini-workout; trying to dissolve a headache, or reflexing the glands for a quick boost of energy.) But for a full reflex session you will work all the reflex points in one foot, and then proceed to work every reflex in the other foot. You will find this routine gives you the best results. You can be sure that you will stimulate every gland, organ, and nerve center of the body when you work the toes and core of one foot completely.

If you learn to give reflex sessions in this way, it will become a habit and you will not find yourself hesitating or fumbling on the feet wondering if you have contacted all the reflexes. A set routine gives you a feeling of calm and confidence which will be quickly noted by your reflex partner, and will save time.

HOW REFLEXES IN THE TOES CORRESPOND TO HEAD AND NECK

Let's review how reflexology brings health to every part of the human body. In Charts B, F, and G you will see how the big toe corresponds to the head, the right side of the head in line with the toe on the right foot, and the left side of the head in line with the toe of the left foot. This alignment is true for the entire body: the left foot has the reflexes to the left side of the body, and the right foot to the right side.

To work the toes, take the left foot in your right hand (or use your left hand if you are left-handed). Take the big toe between the thumb and index finger and go over the whole toe with a gentle pressing-rolling motion. Pay special attention to the pad on the sole of the toe, as this is where the important reflexes to the brain are found.

If the tenderness is in the basal joint near the foot, then it would indicate something wrong in the neck area.

When working on the top of the toe, near the lower edge of the nail, you may find a tender spot. Work the point for a few seconds because this indicates congestion or inflammation in the front area of the head, possibly the teeth or sinuses. (Refer to Chart D.)

After you have reflexed the big toe, rotate it in a circle, first in one direction and then in the opposite. This will have the same effect as rotating the head itself in like manner for a few seconds. It is very relaxing to someone receiving reflexology, as it eases tension in the neck and upper back muscles.

The Brain Is the Nervous System's Headquarters

The body's movements and activities are controlled by the nervous system. Even what we think about, our memories and emotions, as well as our reactions to the external environment, all happen because of the complexity of the electrical network of our nerves.

There are two main parts of the nervous system: the central nervous system (brain, spinal cord and brain stem), which carries messages to the spinal cord and next to the brain; and the peripheral nervous system (nerves that are involuntarily active, which you do not control at will). This nerve network sends it orders apart from the spinal cord and brain; these nerves cause the body to move without brain thought. For example, when you touch something hot, or step on something sharp, your reflex actions work involuntarily, without waiting for a signal from the brain.

Both systems relate to internal glands and organs and cooperate with the body's various systems, such as digestive, circulatory, respiratory, urinary. Even the endocrine glands and reproductive system receive help from this nerve network.

The brain, as the headquarters, is composed of the most complex section of the system (cerebrum, cerebellum, and brain stem). It is connected to the nervous system by the brain stem, and must have a renewed supply of blood and oxygen at all times or the cells will die (such as in the case of a stroke).

The cerebrum is the largest part of the brain. Memory is stored there, as well as ideas. Sensory information goes to the cerebrum and tells the body what to do. It is divided into two parts, and as unusual as it may seem, the right half controls the left side of the body and the left half controls the right side. (See Illustration 8 on page 69)

After a Stroke, Work the Reflex Area on Opposite Side from Body Trauma

When doing reflexology on a person who has suffered a stroke, paralysis, or a disorder affecting the brain or central nervous system, concentrate your reflex work on all pressure points in both big toes, then go back and work the rest of the toes. The cerebrum in the brain controls the opposite side of the body. If a stroke was in the right side of the brain, the left side of the body would suffer the trauma. In this case give extra attention to the toes on the opposite side from the trauma or disturbance. Keep in mind that reflexes in the left foot correspond to the left side of the brain, and those in the right foot to the right side. Success will depend on the reflex receiver's attitude and the extent of brain damage from the stroke.

Reflex Areas to the Brain

To stimulate circulation to the entire head, reflex all points on both big toes, as well as all the other toes. Concentrate on the big toes first, because each has five zones and represents half of the head. Each of the smaller toes is a separate zone, and represents a zonal breakdown of the big toe; work each to *fine tune* its own specific corresponding area of the head and neck.

Following are several techniques that you can use to send renewed energy to the brain. Use one or use them all. Your aim is to improve all mental abilities, including thought patterns and memory.

A. Start at the basal joint of the big toe, and thumb-walk up each zone to the tip. This will include all five zones on the big toe; then do those of each of the other toes, on the sole side of the foot. Repeat procedure on the top and inside of each toe. To work the

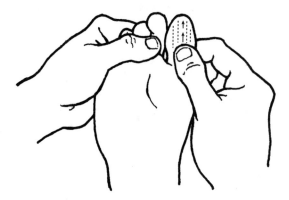

Illustration 20a. Thumb-walk up each zone on the sole side of foot, from basal joint to the tip of each toe. Repeat on the front side of foot. (It may be easier to finger-walk front of toes.) Also work the inside area of each toe by placing index finger and thumb on either side of toe.

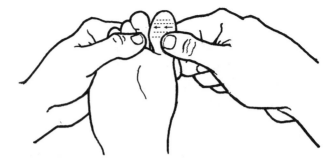

Illustration 20b. Working across each toe, thumb-walk to the left, making several trips across toe; change hands and work across the toe to the right, covering all reflex points.

inside reflex area, place index finger and thumb on opposite sides of each toe; press-and-roll from the tip to the base, and back up on each toe. When you find a sore reflex, focus on it for a few seconds.

B. Of course you can work across each toe if it is easier for you; your purpose is to reach the reflex points under the skin. Use the positions that work best for you.

LOCATING THE HYPOTHALAMUS AND PITUITARY GLAND

You have been learning how to reflex the toes to send a vital life force of energy to various parts of the brain. Now let's get specific. You need to know exactly where the most important reflexes can be found, those to the hypothalamus and pituitary gland in the brain. (Remember that you learned about these very important control centers earlier in the book.)

Many functions of the body are controlled by various hormones; the hypothalamus and pituitary have control over those glands and organs that manufacture these hormones. When giving reflexology to another person, you will want to reflex these very special glands to keep them in perfect balance for good health.

Take the left foot in your hand, and with the top edge of your thumb press into the center of the big toe (see Photo 29). If you have

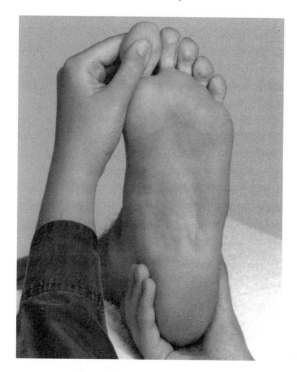

Photo 29. By bending your thumb at the first joint, you can press the upper edge onto the hypothalamus and pituitary reflex points located in the center of each big toe.

studied your charts well, you know that this is the reflex to the hypo-thalamus and pituitary glands which are located in the brain. It will probably be very tender, and you will have to work on it gently at first for not more than a few seconds. Remember to press with a rolling motion. When you go back to it later during the reflex workout, you will find that much of the soreness will have already disappeared.

Next, move your thumb upward just a bit on the toe, and you will be pressing on the reflex to the pineal gland. All these glands are part of the endocrine system, and their potency is beyond compre-hension. Study the endocrine gland chart carefully (Chart E, page 12), and re-read Chapter 25 to learn all you can about these impor-tant glands.

Working the Reflexes to the Neck and Throat

At the base of the big toe you will find the reflexes to the throat and tonsils. Checking for sore spots, work under the pad of the big toe where it is fastened onto the foot to quickly relieve any throat trouble.

I would like to add a note here regarding sore throats and swollen tonsils, which can be caused by various infections. If there is difficulty in swallowing, work the reflexes to the lymphatic system to stimulate lymph fluid. The lymph is a lubricant that carries oxygen to the cells, and also flushes toxins out of the body. When the throat feels dry and hard, like a dry sponge, it needs lymph fluid to soften it and make it flexible again. Work *all around* the base of the big toe, as well as up and down all four sides. It may take several sessions, but in most cases you will find that there will be relief after just one session, and usually during the reflex workout.

Many headaches and eye weaknesses are also caused by tension in the neck area. Keep this in mind as you work on the reflexes of the big toes. If there is tenderness anywhere on the big toe, there probably is tension and congestion in the head, which must be released to promote good health. The outside of the big toe corresponds to the outside of neck, on the same side of body.

Reflexology Benefits for Eyes, Ears, and Sinuses

Eyes ... Windows of the Soul

Now we will move to the next two toes, toes number two and three in zones 2 and 3. To work the reflex to the eyes, place either your thumb, index finger (or a helper tool such as the Reflex Probe) just beneath the second toe, and press with the rolling-pulling motion. Work under the toe and up into the basal joint so that you can reach into any crystalline deposits and break them up. If there is tenderness here, work all the way around the entire toe to stimulate added circulation. Repeat procedure on the third toe, in zone 3.

This reflex work will release a fresh supply of blood to the eyes and will also help open up sinuses.

Refer to Chart F and look at the ten energy zones for a moment. Notice how these zones travel from the toes up through the body to the head (including the index and middle finger on hands, also in zones 2 and 3) on the same side of the body. Study Chart A and notice which glands and organs this invisible energy line passes through. Since the kidney and adrenal are within the same zonal lines, they may be a contributing factor to troubles with the eyes. Also consider working the reflexes of the liver to improve vision problems.

Reflexes to the Ears

Let us now move over to the next two toes, the fourth and fifth (located in zones 4 and 5) which contain the reflex to the ears (see Photo 30). Still holding the foot in the same position, work under these toes (just as you did under the second and third toes for the eyes). Reflex also up into the base of these two toes, as you want to cover the whole area to eliminate any blockages.

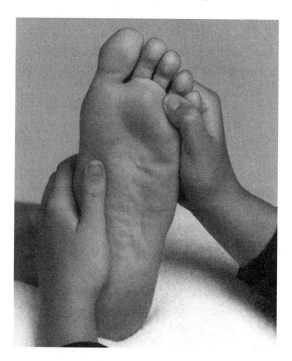

Photo 30. Thumb-walking along the basal joints is ideal for renewing circulation to ears.

Take each toe and press-and-roll all sides, including the basal joints, and work in between toes. Press-and-pull down on the reflex points beneath toes to break up any possible buildup of crystals, to open clogged pathways, and to increase circulation into these important zones.

For middle or inner-ear troubles, also work the reflex area under each toe in zones 2 and 3. To increase stimulation, drop your thumb down just a bit below the eye reflex area and work thoroughly. Search for tender spots, and when you find them, work the area to relieve congestion and improve ear function. (You can suggest to your partner that pulling the ear lobes helps to clear passages of excess fluid, mucous, or wax.) When my husband went to the doctor because of an impacted ear, he cleaned his ear and then advised him on how to keep it free of wax. He told him to use a solution of two or three drops of hydrogen peroxide in each ear to soften the wax, to let it bubble for about one minute, and then to flush it out with lukewarm water from a shower. This should be done once every week to keep the ears wax-free. This is information worth passing on. Also please remember, never poke cotton swabs or any pointed objects into the ears. They

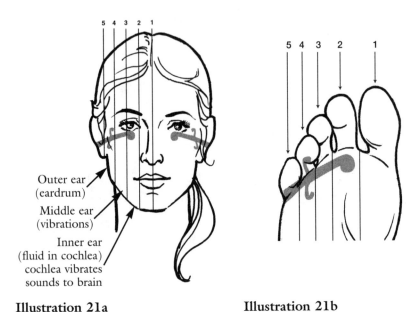

Outer ear
(eardrum)

Middle ear
(vibrations)

Inner ear
(fluid in cochlea)
cochlea vibrates
sounds to brain

Illustration 21a   **Illustration 21b**

could harm the eardrum and the delicate ear bones inside the ear canal.

There exists such a wide spectrum of hearing problems, some of which need medical care, such as arteriosclerosis, middle ear congestion, infections, etc. However, reflexology has been able to relieve many of these problems and has even helped people hear again after a hearing loss.

Remember that taut nerves in the neck can slow down the circulation to the ears in the same way as to the eyes. Always be aware that any tenderness needs to be worked out, because this is congestion signaling for relief.

Helping to Clear Sinus Problems

The sinuses are very small, air-filled cavities in the facial bones, around the nose, on the forehead above the eyes, between the nasal passages, and below the eyes in the cheekbones. When infection occurs, then obstructions or congestion build up, normal drainage cannot occur, and problems result.

To cover all the zones to these areas, work up and down all sides, and the top of both big toes; then work all other toes.

By dropping down immediately below the eye and ear reflexes (which are a little below the second through fourth toes), you will find additional reflexes to the sinuses. Most of these reflex points will benefit from the eye and ear reflex workout as you go over them the first time. However, supplementary stimulation to this area will help to reduce sinus pressure.

Other special reflex points that accomplish wonders in easing the discomforts of sinus congestion are between all toes, but especially between the second and third toes. If your reflex partner is suffering from sinus trouble, you will discover this readily by the extreme tenderness.

Working the tip of each toe sends increased stimulation into each zone to help release sinus congestions. Roll the flat side of your fingernail, top of your finger, or a probe over the top of all toes to help open passageways. You will need to stimulate both sides of the head to relieve sinus discomfort, so work the reflex points on both feet.

Reflexing for sinus troubles gets impressive results; however, it often takes a few sessions for these clogged pathways to clear, and may take a while to bring relief. (Remember, you can suggest that your partner press these same sinus points on the face, and pull the ear lobes to relieve pressure.) You may need to work their reflexes after they have been exposed to irritating substances such as smoke, chemicals, or certain pollens.

How to Reflex for Natural Headache Relief

Almost everybody gets a headache once in a while. There are tension headaches, cluster headaches, sinus headaches, migraine, and vascular headaches, and each one is caused by something different. If one of your friends or loved ones complains of a headache, you know what to do. Have the person sit down and remove shoes and socks. Now it is time for you to use your reflexology skills. You are the best detective in town, and you will find out what is causing the pain.

You know, of course, that emotional stress and poor circulation are two common causes. However, there are many others such as muscle tension, constipation, allergies, sluggish liver, drug toxicity, hormone imbalance, etc.

The first thing you will want to do is relax your partner. Use soft squeezes to the feet, rotate them, and apply pressure to the solar plexus points of both feet. This will feel good and is very relaxing. Both you and your partner should take a few deep breaths for renewed oxygen and then follow a few easy steps for eliminating the headache.

Here again, we will suggest several techniques that you can use to accomplish this. Use only one, or a combination, whatever works best in your situation.

Work the toes first . . . Take the big toe between your fingers and thumb, press into the very center of the pad, searching for the hypothalamus, pituitary, and pineal reflex points. You will be surprised how quickly this will usually work out. If the toe is not sore, then you are in for some additional detective work both to find out what is causing the malfunction and to eliminate it. Check the whole toe for sore spots, and when you find them, work them a few seconds. Check the other toes as well, including the very tips, and end by rotating each toe and each foot.

A special reflex point . . . Work the entire big toe first. Search out tender spots on all four sides and around the base of the toe. You will find a special reflex point that stops many types of headache pain by working on the inside of the second toe just as it joins the foot. Search for it at the basal joint, between the first and second toes, on the top, and on the bottom of each foot. If this is the correct reflex that is telling you of tension causing the head pain, it may be so sore that the reflex receiver will not be able to let you touch it. Search this area between the toes for any tender spots.

Reflex the tips of each toe by rolling the flat part of the thumb nail across the tip of each toe, just as you did to relieve sinus congestion.

To encourage circulation to the head, take one toe at a time between your fingers and stretch it slightly. Never force a toe to move; easy movements are just as effective. As you pull it ever so gently, also rotate it, first clockwise, then counterclockwise, each about three times. See Illustration 6b on page 50.

Rotate top of foot to increase circulation and promote renewed health. Rotating the top of each foot for a few seconds will help alleviate the effects of stress from the body. It relaxes the nervous system, and may release some tense muscles that are causing a headache. Hold the left foot with one hand on the heel, gently rotate top half of foot with the opposite hand. Rotate clockwise and then counterclockwise. Repeat the rotation exercise with the right foot. See Illustration 6a on page 50.

Gently work the reflexes to the spine . . . Working the spinal reflexes will often increase circulation to the head, thus reducing a headache.

As you work each foot remember the importance of the other endocrine glands (the hypothalamus, pituitary, and pineal reflexes already worked in the big toes). After following all the procedures on the toes, work the spine and then down the foot, exploring each gland for tenderness. Work other reflexes, too, including the liver, heart, stomach, and intestines, and find the reflex that is causing the trouble.

Listening to the symptoms will help speed relief. . . A helpful reflexologist will ask a partner what seems to be the matter and will listen carefully to the answer. The information can be a clue to solve the problem (by indicating the reflex areas that correspond to the pain). For example, if your partner tells you of a headache centered at the back of the neck, concentrate on reflexing the sole side of both big toes. Search the basal joints on both the outside and inside edge for sore spots. Also work the reflex area of the cervical spine and surrounding muscle reflexes to reduce stress in the upper spine and shoulder area.

You may be at work when your friend asks you if you could help stop a headache with reflexology. You only have a fifteen-minute break, which is not time enough for a full reflex session, so you must get right to the problem. Ask your friend where it hurts, then proceed to reflex the feet within the same zone, and "listen" to what the reflexes tell you. When these buttons are tender, nature is telling you that this is where the internal trouble lies. This is your opportunity to work the soreness out and free your friend from discomfort.

You can also ask if the person would like to have an eye cover to reduce sensitivity to the light, or a cool, damp washcloth on the back of the neck. Your thoughtfulness will be appreciated. A great reflex-detective *learns to listen for the clues* to bring relief from pain much faster.

Reflexology Is Very Rewarding

Dear Mrs. Carter,

After studying reflexology, I have gained so much confidence and learned to love this kind of work. I enjoy bringing so much relief to people. It makes me feel so good inside, and I am looking forward to helping as many people as possible.

There was one incident that I experienced the other day when I was helping a lady who had some pain in her neck, and had frequent headaches. I started to reflex her feet, and naturally gave the endocrine glands a good workout. Then I came back to the big toe and loosened it up, turned the toe to the left and right. I went on with this procedure for several minutes, until she told me to stop. I stopped, and she said, "You know, something is happening to my neck; the pain is gone, and I believe the headache is slowly disappearing." What a joy for me to hear this! The following day, I gave her another foot reflexology workout, and when I was finished with her, she stood up and walked around the room and said, "It is just like I am walking on air." That made me feel real good. There are so many rewards in this work!

I practice quite a bit of self reflexing on myself, and I am sure that it helps me to stay healthy. When my youngest daughter comes to pay me a visit, she gives me a foot reflex workout, and it feels so good, better than a self-workout. I am amazed how perfect the human body functions, with all the reflexes the Creator has given us. These great reflex buttons help to maintain a healthy condition within the human body.

I want to compliment you, Mrs. Carter, for your tremendous effort in giving us the chance to learn so much about reflexology. I hope to continue your work for the benefit of mankind. For this I thank you from the bottom of my heart.

—J.N., California

CHAPTER 30

Nature Does the Healing

Remember that *you* do not cure any ailment. NATURE does the healing. You merely assist. Through reflexology, nature is able to overcome and throw off congestions and poisons as the renewed strength of the body increases. Reflexology does the job of bringing health and vitality by releasing these forces of nature.

This is possible only if you have mastered your techniques first and are wholly dedicated to giving the best possible reflex workout at all times to transmit the benefits of your skills and knowledge to others.

ALWAYS GIVE A COMPLETE REFLEX WORKOUT

You must always give your partner a full reflex workout, no matter what the complaint. Remember that a reflexology session means that the whole body is getting stimulated, so that all glands and organs are being put back in harmony with each other. This is not possible without the *complete* reflex session, unblocking nerve impulses to *all* organs and glands to normalize and balance the *whole body*.

Of course, there will be exceptions. There may be instances when your partner is in such pain that a complete reflex workout is not possible at the time. In this case, you can use your own judgment and do what you can, giving the complete session later on. Remember that if one part of the body is in malfunction, it has affected other parts which you might least suspect. Never neglect working all the reflexes, if possible, to help your partner achieve a full recovery.

SUCCESSFUL TECHNIQUES FOR RELAXING THE SPINE

You have studied the position of the spine in conjunction with the feet in Chapter 7. Notice in Illustration 9 on page 72 the extraordinary similarity that the inside edge of the foot has to the shape of the spine. Look at Photo 31, and note how to hold the foot with one hand and work the reflex area with the thumb of the opposite hand.

The spine is nature's way to protect the spinal cord and spinal nerves, just as the cranial bones protect the brain. A healthy spine represents the well-being of the entire body.

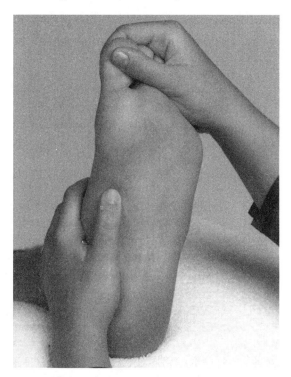

Photo 31. Using the thumb to work the spinal reflex area.

While you still have the left foot in position for reflexing, feel just at the bottom of the large toe where it joins the foot on the medial side. Now move up to its mid joint and this will be the reflex to the top of the cervical spine. Keep in mind that the big toe represents the head and neck.

Notice how the bones of the feet feel like the vertebrae of the spine. Follow these bones down the foot with a rolling-pressing motion as you work vertically down toward the heel. Learn to recognize the upper back reflexes in reflexing the upper part of the foot; then as you continue to work lower, you will find the reflexes to the center of the back. In this way you will be stimulating every vertebra and nerve along the spine as you move downward toward the lower lumbar region.

Now go back and give attention to the sore spots you found on your way down the foot. If your reflex partner is suffering from back problems, you may need to spend quite some time on these tender areas in order to give complete relief from pain.

Never fail to reflex on both sides of the spine to loosen up spinal stress. Work either your thumb or fingers up and down along both sides of the spinal column reflex area. The spine is our tower of strength, which must stay healthy.

Advice for those whom you want to help: in addition to reflexology sessions, avoid putting extra stress on the back by practicing good posture; do not lift heavy items; wear low heels; make sure the bed is firm enough to give the spine its proper support.

Press-and-Roll Between Each Vertebra Reflex

To reach deeply in between each vertebra reflex point, put pressure *across* the spine reflex with your thumb. Start by placing your thumb horizontally across the mid-point of the big toe where the cervical spine reflex starts; press-and-roll the edge of your thumb into this reflex. Move down the toe just a bit, and continue reflexing each vertebra. Work down to the basal joint.

When you get to the seventh cervical reflex, at the base of the big toe, you will feel a bigger bone on the foot. (The seventh cervical vertebra feels like a bigger bone at the back of the neck.) Press-and-roll the edge of your thumb into this vertebra reflex. With the other hand, pull the foot slightly forward, then push it slightly backward. Repeat this procedure down the instep (approximately 26 times, as there are

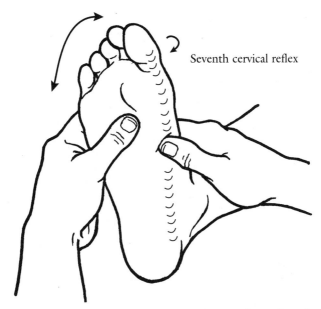

Seventh cervical reflex

Illustration 22. Press-and-roll thumb across vertebrae reflexes found lengthwise on the medial side of each foot. Use other hand to sway foot forward and backward.

26 vertebrae in the spine). Work each vertebra reflex independently until you reach the heel. Remember to do both feet.

The Spinal Twist Reflex

Another very effective procedure to relax the back is called the spinal twist reflex. (See Illustration 23.) Place both hands over the top of the foot; index fingers will be close to each other on the top of the foot, and thumbs will be tucked under the instep, pressing into the spinal reflex area on the sole of the foot. Hold the hand nearer to the ankle in one place, while the other hand gently rocks the foot forward and then backward. Move both hands, still almost touching, and repeat the twisting motion. Feel the thumbs move along the instep of the foot. Start near ankle, continue until you reach the toes, then return back to ankle. This is great for limbering up the spine.

Always work the reflexes of the spine a few minutes each time the foot is worked on. In this way tension on the spinal column and on the whole spinal area is relaxed and muscles cease to contract.

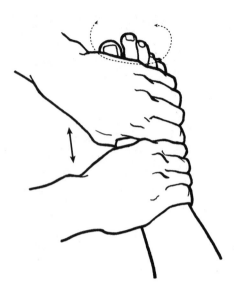

Illustration 23. Position for doing the spinal twist reflex. Fingers are on top of foot, thumbs are against spinal reflex. Helps relax muscles and spine.

Doing this at the beginning of the session will put someone receiving reflexology in a much more relaxed position.

Reflex Stimulation to Skeletal Muscles

Keep in mind there are skeletal muscles attached to the spine which help us to move forward, backward, and sideways. It is very important to keep the circulation moving in these zones. In an average, healthy person, about 30 to 40 percent of the body's weight is in these very necessary muscle tissues. Traditionally a woman has had less muscle tissue than a man. However, today we have many fitness advocates of both sexes who are developing body muscles. There is kickboxing, Tae Kwon Do, karate, and various martial art programs. There is also combat training, self-defense training, and body building. The proportion of skeletal muscles built up in both sexes by participating in these activities is surprising.

It is said that each person has more than 400 skeletal muscles to help the body walk, work, drive, play, cook, eat, etc. Every move we make is controlled by these muscles. This is why exercise is so essen-

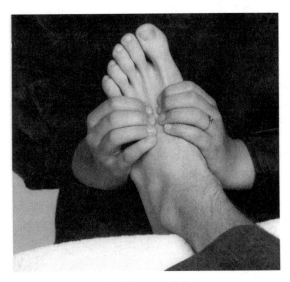

Photo 32. With thumbs on sole of foot and fingers on top, use a very small press-and-roll technique to stimulate the reflex areas on both the top and sole of the foot. This will increase circulation to the skeletal muscles as well as send healing energy to benefit the lymph glands, lungs, vascular system, ribs and chest/mammary glands. Gently work your fingers along each zone.

tial to good health, and why you must use every muscle you can, every day, to keep them strong and healthy.

Work the reflex area all around the spine. This also sends stimulation to many blood vessels and nerves that are housed near that area. Use a considerable (yet not uncomfortable) pressure, and finger-walk from the spine, across the top of the foot, approximately two inches toward the outside edge. Move down the foot covering the full length of the spine.

REFLEXING THE THYROID

Have your reflex partner sit comfortably in a chair with feet raised. You have just finished working the reflexes in the left foot to the spine. Continue to work on this foot until you have covered all its reflexes, before going to the right foot. Move your fingers back to the basal joint of the big toe. Remember, the thyroid gland is located at the base of the neck, so the reflex area will be found at the base of the big toe. Reflex back and forth in this area, and as you find tender spots, give them extra work.

The reflex receiver may feel more of a dull pain in response to reflexing in this area, instead of the sharp pain that may have been felt in the reflexing of previous pressure points. (Reflexes to different parts of the body will signal trouble by various types of sensations, which you will soon learn to recognize as you progress.)

Study your charts and learn the position of the thyroid in the body and also its reflexes. Keep in mind that this is one of the most important endocrine glands that you are stimulating. When reflexing this gland, you are helping to put it into balance with the other endocrine glands.

The thyroid is the metabolic thermostat of the body which must be kept in complete balance; when it is not working normally, the whole body is out of harmony.

Assistant to the Thyroid

There are helper areas for many reflexes on the feet, and the thyroid has one along the edge of zone 1. Reflexing this assistant area helps relax the nerve impulses within the zone and stimulates circulation, helping renew a sluggish thyroid.

Move the thumb from the spine area, near the lower edge of the pad, just beneath the ball of the foot. With a walking, pressing

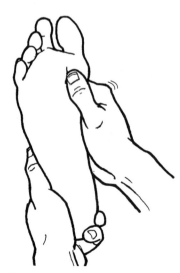

Illustration 24. Assistant reflex to the thyroid.

motion, work the thumb up to the base of the big toe. Remember to press slightly under this pad, as you progress upward toward the lower part of the big toe.

Reflex Top and Bottom of Foot

Your partner may feel weak and fatigued, complain of being cold most of the time, and may have a hard time mentally preparing to do things that need to be done. You can help promote unblocking of any stagnation in the area by reflexing the *top and bottom* of the foot at the same time. This technique provides extra beneficial stimulation.

Rest your partner's foot on its heel. Using both of your hands, apply pressure with fingers and thumbs all around the base of the big toe. Continue to work with fingers on top of foot, and thumb on the sole. Work the outside of zone 1 (toward outside of foot) starting between toes one and two. Press and roll from the base of toes, to just under the ball of foot. Repeat the procedure three or four times. Since this is also the reflex for the bronchial tubes, reflex work in this area will be beneficial in clearing bronchial inflammation.

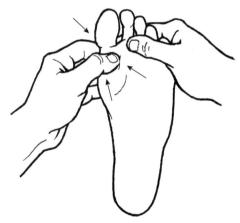

Illustration 25. Assistant position for working top and bottom of thyroid/parthyroid reflex area. Also refex work in this area is beneficial to the bronchial tubes.

Parathyroids

The tiny parathyroids are located just in back of the lobes of the thyroid gland. When working on someone's feet, you will have to dig in fairly deep to stimulate their reflexes. Unless they are very tender, you will not be able to reach them with your thumb, but will have to resort to a tool such as the eraser on a pencil or a hand probe. You may even have to use the pointed end of the probe for this. It will take some experience on your part to tell how deep to press and the right position to use.

If you have no particular reason to think these need special attention, then don't worry about them. They will get the benefit of the reflex work that you give the thyroid, since you can't help but work the parathyroids at the same time.

Remember that this gland is responsible for your reflex partner's poise and tranquility, and many other emotions, as well as physical characteristics.

Thyroid Problems Helped

Dear Mrs. Carter,

As I have used reflexology on myself during the recent years, I have "cured" myself from a crippling arthritis and alleviated a lot of other problems, which pills would not have done. I have also been able to help a lot of my friends and family with great success, including a friend with thyroid problems; within a few weeks she noticed a big difference, making her a believer in reflexology. Life is too short to be spent in misery.

Thank you for sharing your knowledge.

Yours very truly,
—E.L.B.

How to Work the Reflexes to the Lungs, Bronchial Tubes, and Thymus

Note in Chart B how the lung reflex lies along the pad under the little toes. While holding the left foot firmly with the left hand, use your right thumb to work along this pad just under the toes with a pressing "walking" motion. This is a large reflex area to cover; therefore you will need to make several paths over the pad. You can also choose from a variety of reflex techniques to use here. You have just learned to thumb-walk straight across the whole pad.

Criss-Cross Technique

You can also use the right hand to support the left foot, and use your left thumb to work back across the foot, in the criss-cross technique. In this way you will be sure to cover thoroughly all of the reflexes connected with the respiratory system. Cover the whole area; remember you are reflexing more than just the lungs. This workout will affect all the organs within the chest area.

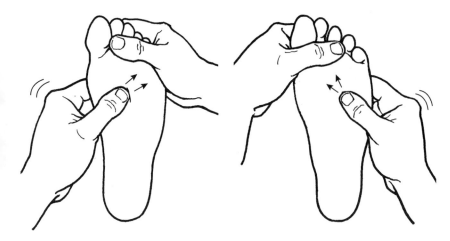

A. Thumb-walk diagonally from instep of foot up to the little toe.

B. Thumb-walk diagonally from the outside of foot up toward the big toe.

Illustration 26. Using the criss-cross technique to work diagonally in both directions across the lung, bronchial, and chest reflex area.

Cough Stopped and Sleep Improved

Dear Mrs. Carter,

I have had a bad bronchial condition for years, caused by "bug spray" being blown back in my face and I inhaled quite a bit, which has caused me to have a very bad cough, both night and day . . . would wake me up at about 3 A.M. One morning I got the reflexology book, looked up the right pressure points, used them, drank a bit of honey-vinegar tea, went back to bed and slept for seven hours,

without a cough, amazing!!! This book has already been
well worth the price.

Thank You,
—M.E.R.

THUMB-AND-FINGER-PRESS TECHNIQUE

You can help boost the effects of stimulation to the lungs and
bronchial tubes, as you did for the thyroid, by working both the top
and the bottom of the foot at the same time. Position your thumbs on
the bottom of the foot, and your fingers on top; with a press-and-roll
movement, work both the top and sole of the foot simultaneously,
covering the complete reflex area.

*Note: Only one of these techniques is necessary for each reflex work-
out session.*

The Thymus Guards Against Infection

The thymus gland has been found to be more important than was at
first suspected by medical researchers. It is quite large in the young
child but diminishes in size as the child reaches puberty. It was once
thought to be useless, but studies have now shown that in young
babies this endocrine gland manufactures master lymph cells that trigger a response of immunity against invaders. These very important
antigen-recognizing cells are distributed to the spleen, lymph nodes
and to the bone marrow to protect the child from diseases, and are
responsible for development of the immune system. If the thymus is
not functioning as it should, the child is susceptible to illness. Later in
life other organs do the job (thymus works in a much smaller degree)
of producing the lymphocytes, which trigger the immune reaction
against harmful invaders.

Sending the life forces to this endocrine gland and supplying it
with the vital energy that it needs by stimulating the reflex may help
it regain its viable role of fighting off the agents of disease. It could
save the life of a child, or maybe even of an adult.

You will see on Chart E of the endocrine glands that the thymus
is located just about where the lung reflex is. Therefore, when you
work the reflexes in this part of the feet, you will also be working the
reflexes to the thymus. No extra reflex work should be necessary for
this gland unless there is definite malfunction.

How to Reflex the Breast/Chest Area

Here again, you can reflex either the top of the foot, the sole, or both, to open up the channels for the vital flow of energy needed to unblock lymph nodes and help equalize tissues of the mammary glands.

To work the top of the foot, support it in the same way, only use your index finger to "walk" between all the metatarsal bones on top of the foot. (These are the five long bones from end of toes to about the middle of the foot. See Chart I.)

Start between the big toe and the second toe, and by "walking" between the metatarsals, travel about three inches toward the leg. The breast/chest reflexes will be covered when you reflex the lungs. Detailed techniques and gentle reflex methods of stimulating energy to release clogged toxins and mucous from the mammary glands can be found in Chapter 33.

Reflexing for the Diaphragm

The diaphragm is a sheet of muscle that stretches from mid spine to the front of the body, under the lungs and ribs above the abdominal area. You most likely have learned how to use the Heimlich Maneuver so

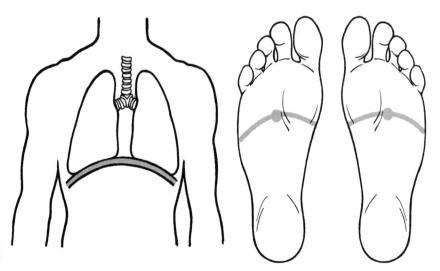

Illustration 27a. Location of diaphragm beneath the lungs.

Illustration 27b. Location of diaphragm and solar plexus network reflexes on the bottom of feet.

that in an emergency you would be able to help a choking victim eject an object which has stuck in the throat. (In this maneuver you place your tightened fist just below the diaphragm to start the procedure.)

It is also this special diaphragm body-reflex-point (located at the mid-base of the ribs) that you can press and hold to stop the involuntary contractions of hiccups.

Since the lungs do not have muscles, the diaphragm helps them out by contracting and then relaxing, thereby making room for their air. When a person is breathing quietly, the diaphragm shifts about an inch; however, when a person becomes energetic, and breathing becomes deeper, the floor of the diaphragm will move up and down about three or four inches.

Since the diaphragm stretches across the body, its reflex area will be found across both feet (see Illustrations 27a and 27b). To work this reflex, place your thumb at the instep of the foot and follow the contour of the ball of the foot across to the outside. As you reach the very center-point of this reflex the solar plexus, press in and hold for a few moments. At this time you can have your reflex partner take in a deep breath and then, as you release the pressure, slowly exhale.

Reflexing Across the Solar Plexus

The solar plexus is a network of nerves that is centered in the upper torso of the body. By studying your charts you can see this reflex is situated in the center of the foot. The complex of interlacing nerves is situated behind the stomach and in front of the diaphragm. You have already stimulated energy through the neurological pathways of the solar plexus as you worked the diaphragm in the same zone areas.

You should keep in mind that working *slowly* over this web of crisscrossing nerves in this reflex area of the foot is a very relaxing procedure, which may cause the reflex receiver to fall asleep.

There is a solar plexus reflex point in the center of *each foot*. Use both hands to press these points to decrease anxiety and nervousness. The technique of using two thumbs to work this reflex in both feet at the same time is very beneficial, and a little different from the press-and-roll, or "walking" method that we have been doing. This procedure is often used for relaxation at the beginning and/or end of a reflex session, because it's wonderful for relieving stress and tension. (You can also use it now, in the middle of the workout, but do not

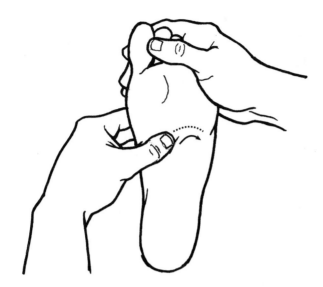

Illustration 27c. Walking the thumb across the diaphragm and solar plexus reflexes on the left foot.

overdo during any one session.) See Photo 38, on page 305, and notice the position for holding the thumbs on the solar plexus points of both feet. Working *quickly* over this reflex area is often revitalizing to the whole body.

Give Nature a Chance

Learn the position of every reflex to every part of the body. Learn how to use your thumbs and fingers, or a self-help tool if one is needed, to release the vital life forces back into the part of the body which the reflexes tell you need help.

Remember, the body is self-repairing, self-cleansing, and self-healing, if given half a chance. And this is what you are doing with reflexology . . . opening up clogged and closed channels so that nature can move in and restore the system to normalcy.

Developing a Special Touch

While you are doing reflexology, keep in mind that this is a special technique that will tell you which organs or glands are not functioning perfectly. Then it is up to you to decide what is really causing the trouble so that you can concentrate on this area. At first you will not be able to do it easily, but with experience it will become second nature as you cover the feet with your healing fingers. It isn't so important that you be able to tell just what is causing the health problem of the receiver as it is to be able to find each tender spot on the feet.

This will be your signal that there is congestion and trouble in whatever area the reflex corresponds to. Concentrate on working all the tenderness out. NOT ALL AT ONCE, of course . . . just remember where the sorest spots are, so that you can return to them later for a little extra reflexing.

WORKING THE STOMACH REFLEX

The stomach is of great importance to the well being of the whole body. In some parts of the world, such as Central Mongolia and Tahiti, natives have the custom of removing shoes before eating, as they feel this aids digestion. As remote as this may sound, there is an

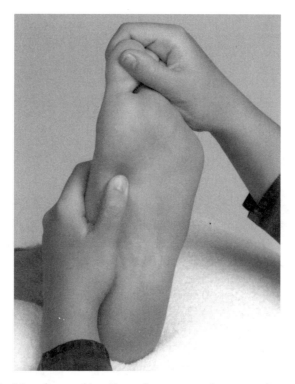

Photo 33. Position for working the reflex area to the stomach, pancreas, and duodenum. Working the soft tissue in the upper arch of each foot is helpful in stopping many digestive troubles.

association between the feet and the stomach. Interestingly enough, those who have sore or tired feet often complain of loss of appetite and abdominal disorders. After a few reflexology sessions (usually only one makes a difference), the abdominal distress disappears and a natural appetite returns. So you see, foot comfort and relaxation may well be related to a healthy digestive system.

To work this reflex, hold the receiver's left foot with your right hand. With the thumb of the opposite hand, press very gently on the soft indented area under the pad in zone 1.

Start reflexing the stomach area by placing your thumb right over the spine reflex. Slowly walk your thumb toward the center of the foot and continue to work across the foot into zone 3. Or you can work the stomach reflex by slanting your thumb a bit, and walking it diagonally in the direction of the little toe; change hands and work back down. Use moderate pressure and do not work too long here, as this reflex may be very tender at first. Be aware that its overstimulation can cause the receiver to feel nauseated.

Notice the hard tendon which leads from the big toe down the foot. This should not interfere with your work. If it is extremely tight, bend the receiver's toes toward you a bit to relax the tension.

When giving yourself reflexology, it is easy to judge the amount of pressure to use; however, when reflexing another person, it is up to you to find out just how much pressure can be tolerated without too much discomfort.

Continue working this area back and forth, remembering that the stomach does cover quite a large area. Don't work down into the waistline of the foot, because this will be getting too close to the kidney reflexes, and these will need special attention later on.

This may sound like a lot to learn, but you will be surprised at how soon all of this will become second nature to you. You will *feel* what the receiver needs, and be able to help restore renewed health.

Reflexing the Pancreas

Since the stomach and pancreas lie so close together, the pancreas reflex will be thoroughly stimulated as you work the stomach reflexes (and later on as well when you reflex the kidneys). Continue to press and roll your thumb almost entirely across the foot.

Remember that here again we are dealing with one of the endocrine glands. The pancreas has a dual activity, and functions as both an endocrine and exocrine organ. (Read more about the pancreas in Chapter 25.) This particular gland is the maker of insulin, so always warn the reflex receiver that reflex work may cause an increase in the natural flow of insulin, usually by encouraging a balance of blood sugar levels. Make this particularly clear if he or she is diabetic and is taking insulin, because intake of insulin may have to be adjusted.

Mastering the Reflexes to the Heart and Arteries

Next you will learn to work on the reflexes to the heart. No one will deny that this is *the* important organ of the body. When the heart is malfunctioning, the whole body is thrown out of harmony; if not corrected, death will occur, or one will live a half-life of suffering and misery. This all sounds very grim; however, each of us has the opportunity to help our body maintain its well-being. If this can be done by promoting stimuli in a natural self-help manner, let it be done. Use reflexology to balance the body naturally and, through the wonder of nature, normalize a healthy heart and circulatory system.

Since learning about the heart is very important, you might like to go to the library for a book on the human body. As you study this powerful little muscle pump, you will be amazed at how uniquely it functions. The main thing to keep in mind is that you are going to learn how to work its reflexes to release any and all congestion both in the heart, as well as in the surrounding arteries and veins.

Notice in Chart A, how the heart is located behind the breastbone, between the lungs. Yet the reflex chart shows the reflexes to be more prevalent on the left side of the left foot, even covering the pad under the little toe.

The heart requires blood vessels to carry blood to it through veins. The veins on the left carry blood from the lungs, and are full of fresh oxygen. This blood is pumped through the left ventricle into the

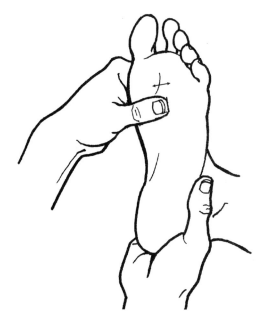

Illustration 28. Working across chest reflex area to benefit the heart, arteries and veins. Work the left foot from the chest to the shoulder reflex area to include the pulmonary artery and veins. Good circulation is critical to the performance of the heart.

heart. After circulating through the body, blood that has less oxygen returns to the heart on the right side. Stimulation to these reflexes will boost nature's energy, giving the cardiovascular system a better chance to fight off heart disease.

Working the Circulatory System

Let us start working on the reflex to the heart by getting into position. Take the left foot in your hand; use your thumb to walk across the chest area reflex to the shoulder reflex. This whole area must be reflexed thoroughly. If you are working on a person who has heart trouble, then search carefully in these areas for pinpointed sore spots, working from the center of foot, clear across to outside, including the little toe and on top of the foot.

To send energy to the heart and circulatory system most effectively, work clear across the whole chest reflex area. Most chest reflexes will be covered (on both left and right feet) while you are reflexing the lungs, diaphragm, solar plexus, and stomach; that is, except those in zones 4 and 5, especially important in the left foot, so give them extra attention. Your goal, remember, is to send nature's vital energy through the pathways to the arteries and veins in order to benefit circulation and discourage clogging.

We can compare the heart, veins, and arteries to the engine of a car. They must be in top working condition to keep the heart pumping needed circulation throughout the body, just as gas and oil lines in a car must be kept sludge-free to keep the engine running smoothly.

When the Heart Doesn't Receive Enough Blood —Angina Pectoris

Occasionally after stress or exertion (especially for those who overeat or smoke) there is an increased demand placed on the heart by the body. When the heart cannot get the needed amount of blood fast enough, the body slows down its mechanism so that the heart's demand for blood can be met. This is referred to as angina, identifiable by a dull suffocating pain in the center of chest. Pain can also be triggered in the upper abdomen, up into the neck, and down the arm into the little finger.

The Importance of a Complete Reflex Workout

Keep in mind that many times the heart may have quit because of the malfunction of other faulty glands or organs. When one gland does not hold up its part of the body's teamwork, it disturbs the harmony of all the interrelated systems. This is one of the reasons why it is so important to work every reflex to every part of the body. Then no congested organ can cause another part of the body to deteriorate and even stop.

Prevention of Heart Trouble

The heart is the most important muscle a person has, so use all the preventive measures possible. We need to use it, as muscles must be used or they lose their strength, but take care never to overdo; *proper* exercise is the way to go for good health.

You can also suggest that a person self-help by altering lifestyle. What can one do?

1. Stop cigarette smoking, as nicotine speeds up the heart rate.
2. Exercise to keep blood pressure down by walking 20 or 30 minutes, five or more days a week.
3. Watch one's diet by eating low-fat foods and cutting back on salts to help reduce weight and cholesterol.
4. Use reflexology to increase circulation throughout the entire body.
5. Stress will contribute to heart troubles, so remember to stimulate all reflexes that relax the whole body. Never forget that rest and complete relaxation are very important to a healthy heart.

If someone you know needs additional help, refer to Chapter 15, pg 122, and read "Prevention Is the Key to a Strong and Healthy Cardiovascular System."

THE SPLEEN

The spleen, like the thymus, is made of lymph tissue, and is part of the lymphatic system which helps filter out foreign matter and flush it from the body. It is the biggest mass of lymphatic tissue within the body. The spleen destroys worn-out blood cells, and stores healthy ones; it actually serves as a storehouse for iron needed by the blood.

Locating the Spleen Reflex

Refer to Chart B to locate the reflex to this important gland. Take the left foot in the right hand in the same position you used for working the reflexes to the stomach (see Photo 33, page 255). Walk your thumb across the foot, from the stomach reflex to the spleen reflex; then work this point with a rolling motion and press in deeper on every third roll of your thumb.

You will notice that this area, as well as that of the liver reflex on the right foot, is quite tender if the receiver is anemic. Give extra attention to both, as well as to the lymphatic system reflex areas. Pump the feet back and forth, or suggest that the receiver do it to help stimulate lymph flow.

ADRENAL GLANDS

The adrenal glands are part of the all-important endocrine system. These two small glands are critical to normal body functions. Each adrenal gland sits on top of a kidney, and each has two parts. The inner section (medulla) makes hormones, such as adrenaline, that work with your nervous system. These hormones help speed up metabolism to help a person react to fear or anger, and are responsible for additional strength in times of emergencies.

The outer section (cortex) of the gland makes hormones that regulate the body's metabolism of foods and liquids, including fats, carbohydrates, sugars, and proteins. When these hormones are out of balance one can suffer from fatigue, poor memory, moodiness, poor circulation, and a craving for sweets which can result in diabetes or hypoglycemia. Some steroid drugs are harmful to the adrenal glands. Realizing the delicate interrelation between the glandular system and organs will make you more zealous to learn where the reflexes are located and how to apply reflexology effectively.

How to Reflex the Adrenals

Hold the left foot in position with the right hand and note how the thumb of the left hand is held. Instead of laying it across the foot as we did previously, place it in an upright position. In this way, you can readily see that the thumb is placed right in the reflex area of the left kidney. Now move the thumb up just a little toward the toes, and slightly to the inside edge of the foot, and you will be on the reflex to the left adrenal gland.

Now with your thumb in this vertical position press in with the top edge of your thumb. Press in and pull downward slightly with your thumb. Holding your thumb on the same point, repeat the press-in-and-down motion about seven times. Be aware that you are working the reflex to the little cap on top of the kidney. As you work with the thumb on the adrenal reflex, be careful not to move into the kidney area; the kidneys are very potent glands and require special care in reflexing.

If you have found the reflex to other endocrine glands extremely tender on this foot, then you will very likely find this adrenal reflex very tender as well. If so, be gentle at first. Remember we are not trying to work out all of the soreness, or cure a condition which has developed over a long period of time in one session, so don't torture your reflex partner. Be patient with nature and with reflexology.

Nature will never fail you; it will only truly amaze you many times with the marvelous suddenness with which many illnesses are healed. Yes, in some cases, with only one reflex session! But not everyone is the same. Each person is an individual, and must be treated so.

Reflexology Affects the Whole Body

Dear Mrs. Carter,

I have been aware of the function of the adrenal glands for some time, knowing that they should produce adrenaline, and more in cases of emergency. What I did not realize was that it was possible to improve this function with a little help from reflexology.

My life has been filled with one trauma after another. My doctor treated me with muscle relaxants and nerve pills. My chiropractor told me that my adrenaline supply had been exhausted long ago because of overwork. His treatments did help but not permanently. Now I am working on the cause of the problem.

I marvel at the complexity of God's great creation and His bountiful provisions for taking care of the body, or the means of bringing it back to health, if neglected. The vastness, yet the simplicity of the whole "reflexology therapy," with ALL of its healing virtues, affects one's health and well being. I discovered that there are many opportunities throughout the day to reflex the feet and the hands.

The over-all purpose of reflexology is its interrelation to ALL body parts. I realize the importance of the WHOLE BODY, or person, and the value of really caring, and giving of one's self.

—F.M.

WORKING THE KIDNEY REFLEXES

Stay in the same position as for working the adrenal gland, with the thumb still in a vertical position in the center of the foot. If the functions of the kidneys are not clear in your mind, refer to Chapter 12 to refresh your memory; see also Charts A and B for their location and reflexes.

Keeping in mind that the kidneys are the body's chief organs for cleansing its internal fluids, let us do all we can to keep them healthy and in perfect balance, so that they can perform normally. They are located behind the abdomen and give the appearance of being positioned lengthwise, one on each side of the spine. Each is about four inches long and bean-shaped. It is interesting that the reflex to the kidney is about the size and shape of a "kidney bean" and lies lengthwise, one on each foot, over to the side of the spine reflex.

The kidney reflex can be one of the most painful of all reflexes. Be aware that you can also make the receiver ill if you work too long or press too hard when it is very sore. Use great caution here, especially when you are working someone's feet for the first time.

Now with a rolling-pressing motion, we will work the kidney reflex. Press the right thumb just below the adrenal reflex, and toward the center of the foot a bit, and work on down to the reflex of the colon, or the waistline of the foot. In some cases you may find a raised place in this area about the size of the kidney reflex; then you will know that the kidney needs help in rebuilding itself, and you will use the natural method of reflexology to give it this boost.

As you work this reflex, watch the expression on your partner's face. If it is too pained, quit working and go back later. The reflex may stay tender for several sessions, so take care not to overwork this spot in any single session. Space the sessions to every other day at first. Offer your partner extra drinking water before each workout, and give nature time to flush out the toxins.

Kidney Stones

If there is a problem such as kidney stones or gout, reflex the entire urinary system. In the case of kidney stones, calcium deposits or tiny stones may get lodged in one of the ureters and cause severe pain, so reflex the ureter tube several times.

Start with the thumb in a vertical position in the center of the foot. With a rolling-pressing motion, work the kidney reflex. Then "walk" your thumb down the reflex of the ureter tube, and work the bladder reflex. Now you will reverse hands and "walk" the opposite thumb up the tube, following it up to the kidney reflex. You may need to work back and forth on the ureter tubes of both feet several times. (See Illustration 14, page 99.)

Also work the lower spine reflexes, as the lower back will have a dull ache. Other symptoms of kidney stones are fever and vomiting, painful urination, a feeling of strong cramps on one side, or pains in one hip and urinary tract. Kidney stones are very painful. If your family is prone to them, improve diet, exercise and use reflexology, as stones are preventable with some dedicated effort.

Gout

Victims of gout often suffer agonizing pain in the big toe due to a metabolic disorder which causes uric acid deposits to accumulate in the joints. Little crystals trigger a painful response, sometimes causing degeneration of the bone. Work the reflex to the kidneys which filter out impurities and clean the blood of waste materials.

Work all reflexes to the urinary system, as this will help filter out inorganic mineral waste and clean the blood. Always send energy to the liver by working its reflex area because it, too, is a great filter.

Also work the body-reflex-area or the referral area, which would be the joints in the thumb or finger in same zone, on same hand. (Refer to Chart F.) A complete reflex workout will help the whole body break up and flush out uric acid from the blood and tissues.

How to Use Reflexology to Help Others Maintain Good Health

Reflexology is a blessing, and is an easy way to maintain good health. It is a comprehensive in-home therapy that can be used by almost anyone to help one's self and others to a greater level of health. It is a natural wonder, and is being used by many doctors in their rehabilitation programs. Proven beyond a doubt to have incredible powers for renewing health to the whole system, both physically and mentally, reflexology is being used successfully as a natural and drugless method of preventive health care.

Good health is the reflection of how one chooses to live one's life. Many people suffer needlessly and silently from ailments in the alimentary canal, or digestive tract, and especially in the lower portion of the route along which waste material from food passes. The colon is very important in maintaining good health; however, it is often neglected until the body's orderly functions are disrupted. Yet when reflexology is used to recognize the "signals" of a disorder, proper stimulation to these signs (sore spots) will help correct the true nature of an illness or disturbance before it becomes serious.

The Intestines

The intestines are divided into two parts, the small narrower section and the large wider section. Notice in Chart A how the large intestine (also known as the colon or bowel) makes almost a complete circle around the smaller intestine within the abdomen.

The small intestine winds back and forth, then connects at the ileocecal valve and becomes the large intestine. This intestine, therefore, starts on the right side of the body and loops around the smaller one, over to the left side of the body, down to the rectum, where the waste leaves the body. If the intestines were straightened out, together they would reach from twenty-five to thirty feet on the average.

Working the Colon Reflex Area on the Left Foot

It is important to send activating energy to the transverse and descending colon first; just like a hose, nothing will pass through until the blockage is first loosened and removed. Since we are working the left foot, the first part of the colon to receive reflex stimulation will be the transverse colon. Holding the left foot with the right hand under it for support, place the thumb of the left hand at the "waistline" of the foot where it bends (see Photo 34).

With a slow, rolling, or push-in and pull-back motion, work across the foot to the outer side, searching for tender spots all along this area. Try to remember where the sore spots are located as you pass over them so that you may return and give them special attention later on. This is very important and with practice you will soon learn to do this naturally.

Now you have reached the outer edge of the foot. (Notice in Chart B how the colon reflex bends down toward the heel, and back across the heel to the rectum reflex.) Follow this reflex across the foot, down the outer edge of the foot, and then back across to the inside edge of the heel pad. Change hands to get the proper pressure on this long reflex area as it continues its turns from horizontal, to vertical, and back to a horizontal angle. (See Illustration 16, page 132.)

If the person whose reflexes you are working complains of an unhealthy colon, you will want to work back up the reflex area with

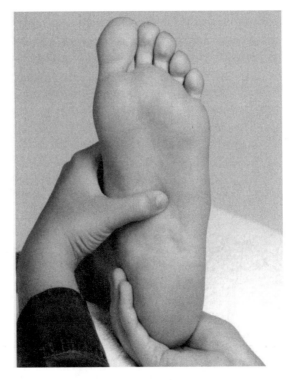

Photo 34. Work the transverse colon reflex just below the waistline of the left foot by thumb-walking across all five zones.

your thumb, or a helpful tool, using the press and pull-down method (see Illustration 5, page 48). Centralize your attention on the sore spots along the way.

Working the Reflex Area of the Small Intestine

Now you have finished working the reflex to the left side of the colon. Let us go on to the small intestine while you still have the left foot in this position. In order to work the reflexes to the intestine, place your thumb vertically or horizontally, just below the reflex to the colon which is on the waistline of the foot. With a rolling-pressing motion, work this whole area down toward the heel and even on down into the heel pad itself. Remember to work the reflexes on the right foot also.

Extra Reflex Help for Elimination Troubles

If the person you are working on has problems with constipation or colon toxicity, some additional reflex attention may be needed. Use the criss-cross technique to cover all the reflexes to the whole lower torso of the body, from the waistline to the pelvic area. Hold the left foot with one hand over the toes for leverage; now tip the top of the foot outward a bit, and reflex with the other hand. Start at the inside-bottom of the foot, and work across the foot in a diagonal angle to the waistline.

Now change hands and alternate directions. Reflex from the waistline to the bottom of the heel on the outside of the foot. You may find new sore spots while working at this angle. Use this technique on the right foot, too.

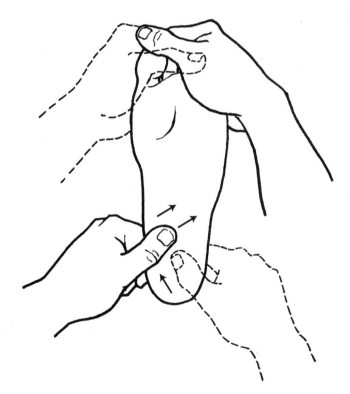

Illustration 29. Work the whole pelvic reflex area by using a criss-cross technique across the heel. Remember to do both feet.

Reflexology Is Totally Awesome

Mrs. Carter,

Health and vitality can be restored through reflexology. For myself, it is giving me a feeling of self-worth. I absolutely love to be able to help people in this way. Reflexology is totally awesome (how it relates to the body, etc.), but at the same time actually simple in that it is drug-free and just helping to aid the body do its natural thing! We are wonderfully made.

The colon is the seat of many illnesses; reflexology is beneficial to unblocking the congestion. Also varicose veins can be helped through working the reflexes of the colon and liver. I am SO HAPPY to be able to learn this technique. If more people were aware of reflexology and tried it, I'm sure a lot of surgery could be avoided! I can't tell you how grateful I am. Thank you, Mildred Carter, I would love to meet you in person! Maybe someday I will.

—Ms. P.F., Alabama

Reflexology Helps Lady Talk and Laugh Again

Dear Mrs. Carter,

I have been so impressed with all your information and success. I have been working with my friend's mother who is in really bad health. Her kidneys no longer function and she has diabetes. She cried a lot and would just lie on the couch and get to where she could sleep, which was most of the time. She would not try to carry on a conversation. She had to have an enema for her bowels to move. I started working on her feet; after seven reflexology sessions, her bowels moved naturally for the first time in a year!!! She still has to have enemas but she also has had several other natural bowel movements.

After I worked on her for two months, she is talking and laughing like her old self. She walks with her walker now and was feeling good enough to get out and go into a department store last Monday. She has not done this in a year! She says "It's the reflexology that helped!"

I also took your advice and encouraged her to walk with her walker and get out of the house with the lady who stays with her. People in this type of condition tend to give up and not want to live. We can have enough influence on people by what we say to them to change their attitudes. An outsider can sometimes do more with a sick person than the family. That's what happened here. It is a great feeling to know that you have helped someone. Her sister cannot believe the difference in her. I pray that the Lord will use me, via reflexology, many more times to help people.

Thank you so very much!
—F.A., Texas

THE BLADDER

There seems to be an alarming number of bladder infections among women. These painful disorders are caused by using the wrong soaps, or by wiping from the back to the front when cleaning genitals after a bowel or bladder movement. Always place your hand behind you and wipe from the front to the back, and keep these areas clean. Teach children this, too. Also keep this area dry, because moisture breeds bacteria. Often infections come from a heavy menstrual flow, tampons, or birth control devices. Other causes are viral infections, venereal diseases, or other bacterial infections.

Women who are susceptible to urinary tract infections should drink lots of healthy liquids, and should make sure they empty their bladder every few hours while they are awake, and always after intercourse.

Men who get bladder infections should also follow the guidelines of drinking lots of healthy juices and water. Check for sore reflexes in the prostate, as well as the whole urinary system.

Anyone infected should stay away from caffeine, carbonated, and alcoholic beverages and all citrus fruits.

Reflexing the Bladder

With the left foot in position, and the right hand giving support, place the thumb in the soft area just below the ankle and instep of the heel pad. You will find a soft spongy area here, likened to the softness of the bladder.

You may want to change positions here and work with the right hand while holding the foot with the left hand. Here again, experiment a little and use whichever position is easiest for you.

Work this whole soft area carefully and gently at first and with a rolling-pressing motion, being careful not to press too deeply. Keep in mind that the bladder reflexes are closer to the surface; if you press too deeply, you will be reaching into the reflexes of the lower lumbar area.

Reaching the Lower Lumbar Region

In Chapters 7 and 30, you learned to reflex the entire spine; however, while you are in this position, we will give the lower lumbar reflexes (which will be the five vertebrae of lower back) some extra attention. This region causes many people considerable distress and pain all their lives, with low back aches and constant disturbance.

To work the lower lumbar region reflex, you may have to use something besides the thumb or finger (such as the Hand Probe or

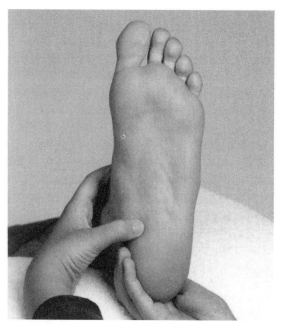

Photo 35. Position for working the bladder and lower lumbar reflexes.

Reflex Roller) to be able to reach in deep enough to reach the reflex. Use the technique that will be most convenient for you, and which will give the best results.

Note on Chart C that the reflex for the lower lumbar is in the same position as that of the bladder.

Place the thumb in the same position that you used to work the bladder reflex. Now move the thumb down toward the heel and a bit closer to the ankle. Press in deeply, as if you were trying to reach through the pelvis to the end of the spine. Stimulation to this area is also beneficial to the nerve supply in the pelvic area, which can help poor conditions of the bladder, as well as constipation and prostate or female problems.

Use a firm, yet even pressure. As in any type of treatment, some pain can be expected by the receiver, but you can keep it to a minimum by taking your time, proceeding carefully and slowly, and then returning to the sore area later on in the session. You will find that each time you reflex this area, it is less painful than the last, so you can work it out little by little.

REFLEX HELP FOR SCIATIC PAIN

If someone in your family has pains across the lower back or radiating through the buttocks and down the thigh, try the sciatic reflex for tenderness. Inflammation in the sciatic nerve will make its reflex extremely tender.

Sciatica is often caused by a ruptured or slipped disk in the lower lumbar (lower back) area. When the injured disk presses against the sciatic nerve, a burning pain radiates through the buttocks and down the thigh.

The two sciatic nerves are the largest nerves in the body, running down each leg from the lower spine, where a network of nerves branches out from it on either side. For this reason you may find that the reflex on one foot is much more tender than the reflex on the other.

Work Both Sides of Spinal Reflex

Since the sciatic nerves come down the spine, you will want to work the spine reflex to make sure there are no pinched nerves. Using both thumbs see Illustration 10 (or with one thumb and index finger), work both sides of the spinal reflex simultaneously. Concentrate on the lower section, working from the waistline down to the heel to send healing forces of nature to all inflamed and congested parts of the lower lumbar region.

Locate the Reflex Where the Sciatic Nerve Crosses the Foot

This reflex point is located in the lower section of the heel. Notice that it is not centered but is slightly down toward the lower edge of the heel pad. This particular reflex point corresponds to the sciatic nerve pressure point in the buttock. This is where a doctor pokes a finger, checking for a tender reflex in the sciatic nerve. Pressure on this point can cause a severe sharp pain.

One does not need to use deep pressure in the buttock to feel pain. However, the sciatic reflex in the heel usually does require deep pressure to find tenderness. If this reflex is hard to locate, you may have to use a reflex tool that will penetrate more deeply than you can with the thumb. You may have to search for this until you have experience; time and practice will help you find it on the first try. (See Photo 25 on page 157.)

When you have located the sciatic reflex, work it with a deep rolling motion, unless it is too painful. Then ease up and press very gently until you have worked some of the tenderness out.

Work Between the Hip and Buttock Reflexes

Refer to your charts to refresh your memory of the sciatic reflex areas. Start on the instep of the foot and thumb-walk across the foot, working over the point where the nerve crosses the heel, and on across the buttock reflex to the outside of the foot.

Also work around the outside of the foot, and up toward the top a bit to cover the hip reflex. This will be tender if there are painful nerves in the hip (refer to Illustration 36 on page 288).

A. Reflexing the Cord on the Back of Leg

The path of the sciatic nerve branches out and travels down the thigh, past the knee, and into the foot. Move just above the heel, and take the Achilles tendon between the fingers and thumb; work this with a pressing-rolling-motion from the heel on up to the calf of the leg.

B. Reflexing Up the Inside of Leg and Knee

Now with a gentle pressure work up toward the knee, rolling the edge of the leg bone as you proceed; you will probably come across several very tender spots.

When you get to the knee, follow on around it with the same pressing method. In doing this, it will be best to work the whole knee area, around the upper part of the knee and also the underside, thus helping to relieve painful nerve impulses.

Do not use any tools except the fingers while searching out these tender spots in another person's leg. Always be sensitive to the comfort boundaries of anyone you reflex. If you have found many very tender spots here, it can be helpful to relax your partner by slowly rotating the foot. Hold the heel in one hand and gently rotate the foot in a circle four times, stop, then slowly rotate it in the opposite direction four times. This will help promote relaxation, stimulate the lymphatic system, and benefit the flow of circulation for faster relief of pain.

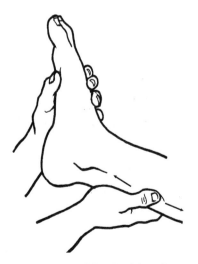

Illustration 30a. Position for working the Achilles tendon.

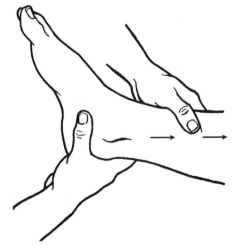

Illustration 30b. Position for working up the inside of leg.

Sciatic Pain Relieved in a Few Days

Dear Mrs. Carter,

I am constantly impressed by the evident interrelatedness of the parts of the body, and therefore of their reflexes. I am personally grateful for having learned (some weeks ago) of the "extended" treatment for the sciatic nerve. I had had such excruciating (chronic) pain in the arch of my right foot, both top and bottom (practically my whole foot!) that I could hardly walk or sleep. I had done the "end sciatic reflex" in the heel for some time to no avail. But when I learned to extend the reflex workout up the leg and into the back, I was relieved in a few days. I resumed my fitness exercises, including a four-mile, four-times-a-week walk!

Blessings,
—M.F.

REFLEX PRESCRIPTION FOR HEMORRHOIDS

Hemorrhoids are one of the most painful conditions and often recur even after three or four surgical operations. Yet the simple treatment of reflexology has stopped this pain, usually suffered in secret, many times after only one reflex workout. And if reflexology is used correctly as a preventative program, hemorrhoids will vanish completely, never to return. However, if there is profuse bleeding which does not clear up in two or three reflex sessions, then you must insist that the person go to a medical care provider to make sure that there is not a more serious problem than you can handle with reflexology.

Working the Reflexes to Dissolve Hemorrhoids

Hold the left foot with the right hand for leverage; using the left hand, place your thumb and finger on the heel of the foot, and start working the bony part. The reflexes go all the way around the heel. They are mostly on the bony structure just above the inside heel pad but don't stop there.

You are searching for a very tender spot and you might find it up toward the ankle or just down from the lower lumbar reflex. Since this represents the inside of the rectum, remember that the congested veins could be internal or external or there might be several veins that are congested. It is up to you to search out the tender reflexes. This may take a little time, but once you find the right spot, you will have little trouble bringing quick relief to the reflex receiver, and it will be lasting.

When you find the correct reflex, work it for a few moments. If there is more than one tender spot, be sure to work them all with the pressing-rolling motion of the fingers. You might even show your partner where the spot is for self-help if necessary.

Many times the hemorrhoids will only be on one side; however, it is best to use the same procedure on both feet. (You may want to wait until you are working on the right foot, but do not neglect this reflex . . . especially if it is tender on the left foot.)

Supportive Reflex to Stop Hemorrhoid Pain

To bring about healing energy and improve circulation to the lower torso and pelvic region, move to the cord on the back of the leg and work this area as you did for the sciatic nerve. Use the thumb and fingers to press and work as you reflex your way up and down the cord; take time to do this thoroughly, and be sure to do both legs.

You will note on Chart C that this cord behind the leg covers the reflexes to several important parts of the body. *Note:* Keep in mind that you do not have to work this area for each separate reflex routine. *One good reflex of the cord on each leg is sufficient for each session.* The procedures given are to help explain individual reflex techniques so that you can readily tell where to work for a specific case of congestion in any certain area.

Take Time for Reflexology

Millions of precious hours and dollars are spent every year on improving the body's outward form and appearance. We appreciate the importance of looking fabulous, but let's not overlook the importance of *feeling* fabulous, too. How many people take the time to understand the inner structure of the human body and all its wondrous functions? Often new mothers- and fathers-to-be take time to read about the incredible efficiency of the body while a new life is forming within. However, once the baby is born, their interests take them elsewhere.

Our bodies may be predetermined by DNA-coded instructions from our heritage, by the environment we live in, and by time. However, if we would spend only a few minutes each day stimulating the reflexes in our (or each other's) feet, we could immensely improve the circulation that carries the much needed oxygen and nutrients to our living cells. We would be giving the body renewed energy to fight off sickness and disease. So don't forget to take time for reflexology; the rewards of better mental and physical health are significant.

How to Use Reflexology to Improve Sex Glands

The reproductive organs go through many changes in a lifetime. At adolescence, the body starts to change inside and outside. For instance, the voice changes, body hair growth increases, and sex organs enlarge.

As a woman ages her body goes through several natural changes such as menstruation, child bearing, and menopause. Men also have both mental and physical body changes during their lifetime. Some of the problems a man may encounter as he gets older are painful ejaculation, urinary difficulties, and oftentimes prostate complications.

Occasionally, both men and women suffer from sexual problems, frigidity, impotence, or sterility. Sometimes a poor diet is to blame; other times the stress and tensions from a busy lifestyle can cause depression or glandular imbalances.

Don't Let Stress Control Your Family's Life

Stress is reported to be the definition of 60 to 75% of all "dis-ease." It is up to each of us to find beneficial ways, such as changing one's lifestyle to include a better diet and improving daily exercise, to cope with stressful situations, as they influence our physical and mental health.

Reflexology is often prescribed (rather than medications) as an antidote for stress. It has been proven to be extremely helpful in reducing as well as preventing stress. Fifteen to twenty minutes a day of reflex therapy helps the body relax and will enhance the body's defense system. It decreases internal tensions and increases emotional stability. Those who use it regularly report fewer headaches and stomach disorders, and claim to suffer less from irritability and fatigue.

Start a Preventive Health Care Plan

Improve the diet of those in your household by making wise decisions about the foods you buy and serve. Use foods from the basic food groups, and stay away from processed, chemical, and junk foods. Encourage your family to participate in fun and enjoyable activities. It is good for the circulatory system to do an exercise that requires deeper than average breathing for at least five to ten minutes each day.

Protect the health and well-being of your family with a beneficial feel-good reflex session. Reflexology is a natural therapy that is highly effective in several areas: it helps to reduce stress and tension; it reduces high blood pressure; it encourages blood and lymph flow throughout the body; and it stimulates its self-repairing mechanisms.

Hopefully you and your family are in perfect health; however, it is never too soon to start on a preventive health care plan. You can help each other with the safe and simple use of reflexology. Learning to work the reflex points to the gonads (sex glands) can be very important to the health and vitality of every living being. These are the chief organs of the reproductive system and they influence one's appearance, drives, emotional outlook, and entire personality. The disposition of each individual is adjusted by the healthy (or poor) condition of these vital organs.

You can help your companion achieve a sparkling personality by using reflexology to these very important glands. It is a thrilling experience to find a tender reflex, because it tells you which organ is signalling for help. Then, as you continue to work this reflex, over time you will notice the tenderness disappearing as the recovery period takes place. Now you know that health will be restored to the ailing organ, so that it can do its proper work within the intricate system of the body. All this without the expensive or invasive use of pills, drugs, or surgery!

Reflexology will be useful for the whole family. Teens, men, and women will all benefit from the reflex work described. Any sore reflex points will relate to you where trouble is beginning within the body, thus reducing possible confusion about a painful situation. Moreover, using reflex therapy helps promote a positive attitude toward health, which is beneficial for everyone. Specifically, we will be dealing with an area of reflexes that surrounds the ankle bones, on the inside and outside of both feet.

A HELPFUL GUIDE FOR REFLEXING THE OVARIES (OR TESTES)

To get started, use the reflex guidelines, and make sure you and your partner are comfortable. Go to the outside of the foot and place your thumb in the fleshy part between the ankle bone and the heel. With the press-and-roll technique, reflex this area completely, all around the ankle on the outer side of the foot. Work over to the back of the ankle and underneath it, searching for specific tender spots.

It might be more convenient for you to use two fingers for this particular reflex. Use whichever technique is easiest and most natural for you, and will give your partner the best workout.

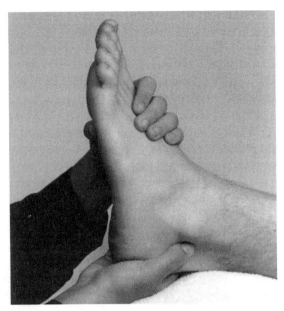

Photo 36. Work the fleshy part under ankle bone and down to the heel on outside of foot, to restore healing circulation to testes on men (or ovaries on women). Reflexes on left foot correspond to gonads (testis or ovary) on left side of body, and right foot to those on right side.

If your partner has any kind of trouble with the ovaries (or testes in men) this area will be extremely sensitive. If you find tender spots, be considerate and very gentle in the beginning, as you do not want to cause much pain. These reflexes can be quite sore, so use a delicate "feather touch" here. Remember to work both feet equally, restoring circulation to both sides of each gland and organ, thus balancing the whole body's state of efficiency.

GUIDELINES FOR REFLEXING THE UTERUS (OR PENIS AND PROSTATE)

Working the reflex to the uterus in women, and those to the penis and prostate in men, is the same. This reflex will be found in zone 1, just under the ankle on the inside of each foot. Gently hold the left foot with the left hand so as not to squeeze. Place the right hand under the heel of the left foot, and with the first two fingers press into the soft area just under the ankle bone. Work all around the ankle on the inside of the foot.

You will probably find that the sorest spot for these reflexes will lie under the ankle bone and back a little toward the heel. Don't fail to reflex all of the ankle area on the inside of the foot just as you covered the outside.

Take care as you use the press-and-roll motion, especially at first. Since these reflexes cover an even more vulnerable area of the sex organs than the reflexes on the outside of the foot, you will have to be doubly careful when starting reflex work here, as it can be very painful. You want to be gentle and not overwork the area. A little stimulation the first few times in this area will accomplish better results for your partner than reflexing too much.

Additional Routine to Help the Gonads

Here is an additional routine for the reflexes below the ankles on the inside, as well as for those on the outside of the foot. As you are holding the foot in position with one hand holding the top of the foot, and

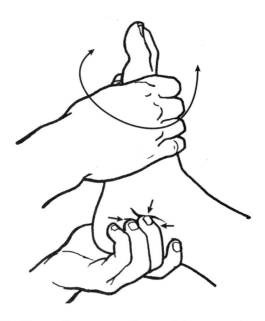

Illustration 31. Rotate foot onto reflexes of the uterus (or penis and prostate) on the inside of foot. Then change hands and place fingers under ankles on outside of foot, rotate foot onto reflexes of the ovaries (or testes).

the fingers from the opposite hand still pressing the reflex under the ankle, rotate the top of the foot to the left four times, then reverse and repeat to the right four times. This sends extra stimulation to the sex glands, and gets the lymph fluids moving to help strengthen the immune system and defend the body against disease. It is a technique you can use as you become more advanced in your reflex work.

Additional Help for the Prostate

Pain or difficulty in passing urine may indicate a swollen or inflamed prostate gland. If the flow of urination is slight and accompanied by a stinging or burning sensation, with symptoms of unusual fatigue, rectal or lower backache and fever, there very well could be a bacterial infection.

Recommendations for natural health care of the prostate include drinking a lot of pure water every day to motivate the flow of urine. Flushing the bladder is important because retention of urine too long can increase the possibility of bacteria in the bladder. These bacteria could then work up the ureters to the kidneys, causing unwanted troubles there.

Eat foods rich in zinc: beans, nuts, raw or steamed vegetables, fresh fruit or fruit juice, and brown rice are a few suggestions. Avoid all fatty, fried, junk, and refined foods. Walking is recommended to increase circulation, as is, of course, reflexology.

When using reflexology, make sure you cover all the reflex points to the endocrine glands, as they are the control centers of the body. Also reflex those to the urinary system, as it is linked with the prostate gland, and those to the lower spine to relieve any tightness in the surrounding area.

You have already given the reflexes to the prostate a fairly good workout on the inside of the foot. When you have completed this work, move your fingers to the back of the foot. It is here that you will begin to work the assistant reflex to the prostate. Start just above the heel, using your finger and thumb; work up the cord in back of the leg, using a pinching-pressing motion as you progress up the calf of the leg. You can bring great relief to those who suffer from disorders of the prostate gland, as it is one of the fastest of the organs to respond to reflexology.

Note: By looking at your charts, you will notice that the reflexes here (cord in back of leg) are to several organs and glands, all located in the lower regions of the body. Use the same technique that you used in reflexing for hemorrhoid problems and also for the sciatic nerve. Review Chapters 21 and 22. Keep in mind that only one good reflex of the cord is necessary for each reflex session.

BREAST/CHEST REFLEX AREAS

All women must protect themselves against lumps in the breasts and mammary glands. If you are giving reflexology to a woman who has been concerned about breast problems, make sure that you reflex the top of both her feet thoroughly to encourage good blood and lymph circulation. Also work the other reproductive glands and organs to release all clogged toxins or mucous formations from the energy pathways. Reflex all the endocrine glands to balance hormone production and the reflex area of the liver to cleanse her system.

Earlier you learned which reflexes correspond to the chest area (Chapter 19). Of course all reflexes are mapped out on the soles of the feet, so working the chest and lung area on the bottom of the feet will benefit circulation to the upper torso of the body, including the breasts. However, the most effective reflex to the breast area is on top of the foot. You will not need much pressure here, as the skin over the top of the foot is very delicate, as is the skin over the breast.

A Gentle Reflex for the Mammary Glands

This gentle method of reflexing the mammary glands is "finger-walking" the top of the foot. Using your supporting hand, hold her foot by the toes and tip it slightly to one side, so that you can see where your fingers are working on the top. With the index and middle finger of the other hand, let your fingers walk the top of the foot, along each zone between the metatarsal bones. Start in zone 1, at the base of the big toe, and work approximately two inches toward the leg. Continue working each zone, ending in zone 5 near the outside edge of the foot. See Illustration 3a in Chapter 5, page 46.

Another beneficial routine is to make small circular movements on the top of each foot, working the same zonal areas between the metatarsal bones. Utilize the method which is most suitable.

Use Two Thumbs to Stimulate Lymph Under the Arms

The breast is made up of milk glands, fat, fibrous tissue, nerves, blood, and lymphatic vessels. There is a large network of lymph glands in the chest area, as well as under the arms. Reflexing the top of the foot will improve the health and circulation of the chest area, and working the reflexes on the outside edge of the foot, on the little toe side, will benefit the lymph under the arms.

Place one hand under the foot and one hand on top. With your thumbs side by side make several very small circles along the outside edge of the foot, from the little toe to the waistline. This will stimulate the lymph reflexes and benefit the lymph circulation under the arms.

A Bit of Friendly Advice

If your companion needs a boost of support, you may want to offer a few helpful suggestions. Many times people know what is good for them, but they may put it out of their minds, or get so busy with life that they forget to take care of what is important . . . their health! Sincere advice is always welcome, and if you are giving your friend reflexology, she will most likely accept other healthful recommendations from you as well.

She should get plenty of exercise (making sure to move her arms as much as possible to generate lymph and blood distribution). She should make sure her diet is nutritious and wholesome, without a lot of sugar, fat, or salt. She should drink a lot of pure clean water to flush out impurities through the elimination of liquid wastes. And she should always use the benefits of reflexology to assist nature in cleaning the body of toxins, promoting internal balance, and revitalizing the health of all living glands and organs.

Dear Mrs. Carter,

Having read about and used many natural healing disciplines, I find your Body Reflexology book most definitely tops them all! God bless, and may you and your daughter be blessed with many more years in which to share this great gift of healing.

Thankfully and with kind regards,
—J.V., Washington

Dear Mrs. Carter,

My very dear friend has shared your book *Body Reflexology; Healing at Your Fingertips* with me recently. I must tell you it has totally changed my life. For six years I have dealt with a body that is not my own anymore. Yet in the short time it took me to read and re-read your marvelous book, my body is now transforming into what it used to be. I give you my heartfelt thanks for this miraculous book of life-saving techniques.

Many, many thanks to you, Mrs. Carter; you have literally saved me from a series of operations, including a total hysterectomy at the age of only thirty-eight.

Gratefully yours,
—B.C., Hong Kong

REFLEXING THE GROIN

As you worked the lower lumbar area, you were also sending vital energy to the groin area and sex glands. If your male partner is having trouble with his sex glands, this reflex area was most likely very tender. Check it again to see if any of the soreness has disappeared; if not, reflex it a few more seconds for effectiveness.

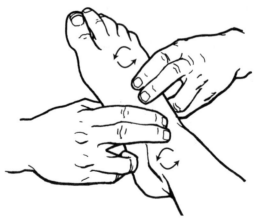

Illustration 32. *Double-Hand Technique* Use fingers with press-and-roll movements over top of foot to stimulate lymphatic system. Also work the reflex area between ankles to benefit circulation of the groin area.

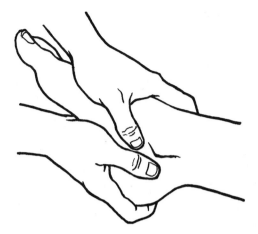

Illustration 33. *Double-Thumb Technique* Place one hand over top of foot, the other hand under the foot. Use both thumbs to gently work the reflex areas of the gonads (under the ankles on the inside, and then on the outside of the foot).

This technique can also be used to encourage lymph circulation. Lace fingers on bottom of the foot, and work both thumbs over the top of foot, from ankle to ankle, and from big toe to little toe.

Working the reflex area from one ankle to the other behind the foot is very beneficial and is especially important for men. Another assistant helper for the groin is to stimulate the lymphatic system on top of the foot between both ankles. Men have many lymph nodes along the ligaments between the pelvis (hip bone) and the medial thighbone (femur on groin side) so stimulation of this area is very valuable.

Men also have several lymph glands in the chest area, as well as under the arms. Work top of foot for chest reflex, and the outside edge of foot, on the little toe side, for the shoulder and hip reflex area.

ACTIVATING THE LYMPHATIC SYSTEM

Learning to work the reflexes to the lymph glands or nodes is very important. These are little clusters of filtering plants along the way of the big vessels of circulation. Unlike the heart, this system does not have a pump to move the lymph along the vessels; only "body motion" keeps this valuable fluid moving. Rotating the foot several times to the left, then to the right, strongly stimulates the lymph glands.

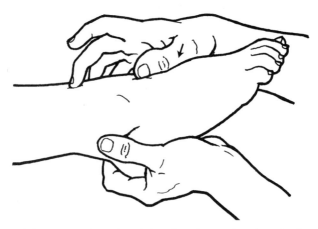

Illustration 34. Using the side of the thumb to stimulate the lymph glands reflex on top of the foot.

You will notice in the illustration how the foot is held while you work the lower lymph reflexes which are located on top of each foot, between the two ankle bones. Note that the reflexes are being worked with the side of the thumb. You may choose to use the end pads of your thumbs or index fingers. Use a pressing-rolling motion across the top of the foot from one ankle to the other.

Another method is to finger-walk over the top of foot, using your index and middle fingers from both hands. Start at the toes and walk your fingers over the top of foot; repeat this several times to cover the full reflex area. See Illustration 3a, page 46. If there is a lot of tenderness in this area you will know that there is inflammation some place in the body. By working the lymph reflexes, you will be sending a surge of the universal life force along the vessels to all of these little filtering plants to help nature eliminate congestion wherever it may be in the body.

HOW TO WORK THE SHOULDER/ELBOW/ ARM REFLEX AREAS

It is best to exercise or rub an aching or stiff shoulder. However, if it has been hurt and is painful to the touch, reflexing the referral area will help stimulate healing circulation. When there is pain in the shoulder, elbow, or arm, it also helps to work the corresponding reflex area to promote healing.

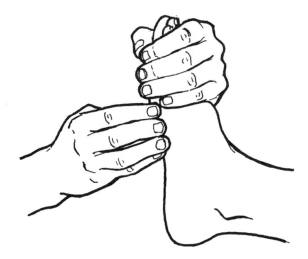

Illustration 35. Working along upper outside edge of left foot to benefit circulation in left shoulder and arm.

Reflex areas on the foot that correlate to the shoulder, elbow, and arm can be found on the outside of both feet; left foot corresponds to the left side, and right foot to right side. The shoulder corresponds to the basal joint of the little toe.

To work these reflex areas, wrap one hand around the foot for support. Keeping the foot upright, use thumb or fingers from opposite hand and work the reflex area from the little toe to waistline and back. (You may feel very small gritty specks under the skin around the basal joint of the toe. These will cause a sharp, painful sensation when reflexed, which signals that circulation is impaired.)

Work along the outside of the foot and up onto the top of the foot a bit. See Illustration 3b page 46. Use a press-and-roll or criss-cross motion to cover the whole region, especially attending to sore points. Increased circulation in zone five will help speed healing energy to the painful section of the shoulder, elbow or arm.

How to Work the Hip/Knee/Leg Reflex Areas

Reflex areas for the hip, knee, and leg are found on the outside of both feet, left foot corresponding to the left side, and right foot to right side. Techniques to use are similar to those for the shoulder/elbow/arm reflex areas. To work, wrap one hand around the foot for

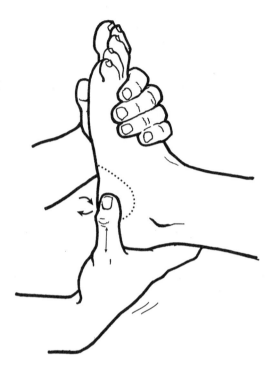

Illustration 36. How to hold the foot and use the thumb to work the reflex areas to the hip, knee, and leg.

support. Keeping the foot upright, use thumb or fingers from opposite hand and work the reflex area from waistline to heel. Work along the outside of the foot and up onto the top of the foot a bit. Use a press-and-roll or criss-cross motion to cover the complete reflex area. Thoroughly work the whole area, concentrating on the sensitive points for beneficial results.

Many suffer pain, aggravation, and sometimes back discomfort from hip, knee, and leg problems. If your partner is having troubles here, work the referral areas. Another reflex for hip pain is the same as that for the sciatic nerve. Work the bottom region in the heel, on sole side of foot. Work from the lower lumbar reflex on the inside, over to the outside of the foot (buttock reflex). See Chapter 22 for techniques of how to work the reflex to the sciatic nerve.

Note: You have worked all the reflexes on the left foot; now it is time to work all the reflexes on the right foot. Always remember to do both feet for best results for the entire body.

When you find a tender spot and you are not sure which reflex it is, work the soreness out anyway. It is telling you that there is trouble some place in the body and it needs your help to loosen the life forces so that nature can take over and do the job of healing.

Rx Stops Leg Pain

Dear Mrs. Carter,

I am 82 years old and a few days ago I fell and hurt my left leg. It was very painful. I took pain pills, but they didn't stop the pain, so I got your Body Reflexology book out and read it. I worked the reflexes and stopped the pain. When I had to be on my feet, my leg would hurt a little, but nothing like it did before. I'd work on the reflexes again; now my leg hardly hurts at all. It's hard to believe anything so simple could do so much good.

Sincerely,
—L.M.B., Oklahoma

Why I Like Reflexology

Mrs. Carter,

I have learned that most things can be cured without medicine or operations by just knowing where to search out and unblock the blockage within the body. My legs sometimes had been yellowish-looking when getting up . . . Thanks to reflexology, now that has gone. I have not seen this yellow color in my legs for a long time now.

I have always believed that the body in which we live during our lifetime is a wonderful part of all things on earth. The body will take care of itself if treated properly; it contains its own defense system towards trouble within. And this is why I like reflexology!

With your help, and God's, it will be O.K.

—R.K.
Illinois

Hello Tammy,

Thank you for your good words, and for being the teacher that you are; at this moment, I salute you as a teacher. We are here to support our friends and guide them, and the feet can help to tell the story of the person's life, like a "short-cut" to finding the problem. Many years back I experienced how good foot reflexology can be and I am convinced of its benefits. Foot reflex was the start for me to begin to pay attention to my body, before damage was done, and I know it will be a benefit to others. I have done foot reflexology on my daughters and husband, and they benefited by it, and sometimes I wonder if even I benefit just as much by doing the reflex work. It feels good to help someone. Foot reflexology is more easily tolerated by many, than a total massage that may just be too much.

As I work on my friend's feet, let me find the way to bring the glow of the light back into his life.

Thank you and sincerely,
—N.B.

CHAPTER 34

Helping Others— One Foot at a Time

Reflexology is nature's "push button" secret for better living, and you are now learning the skills needed to help those who depend on you, primarily your family and close friends. Even if you were to take a trip, or move around the world, you would still retain this ability to help yourself and others with reflexology, one foot at a time.

After you acquire basic knowledge, reflexology will probably come instinctively to you, as this is truly nature's way to relieve pain. In the same natural way that you rub your forehead and neck when they hurt, or twist your hands together when you are nervous, you will develop reflexology skills that will inevitably become part of you. And when someone you know needs to recover from pain or illness, you will be there with your therapeutic touch to provide comfort and give that person a sense of well-being.

REFLEXOLOGY IS WONDERFUL FOR SHARING WITH OTHERS

The first time you administer reflexology to someone's feet, you will be amazed by that person's remarkable feelings when you are done. Perhaps you may hear that his or her feet feel as light as air, or like they have been dancing on a cloud; or maybe the story might be of total relaxation after a stress-filled day.

Since reflexology works from the inside, it helps balance the interplay of all the body's systems, thereby improving the overall functioning of the body. I have had people tell me after a reflex session that they feel as though they've been reborn into a fresh new body. And many have told me that reflexology has actually saved their life.

When performing these important steps of reflexology, remember to affirm kind thoughts of good will toward those you care about. You will be bringing a free-flow of love into action, as the natural forces of nature and harmony work to restore health and renew energy. Reflexology is very rewarding because it brings precious good health to the receiver the natural way. And as the giver of reflexology, you will be repaid with the excitement of witnessing renewed health in those you care about.

Reflexology, Prayer, and Determination Promote Healing

Dear Mrs. Carter,

I have been having some very wonderful experiences using reflexology. I have worked on a serious diabetic who had been diagnosed with tetanus; after reflexology he can eat more, has put on some pounds, his blood sugar level is much better and in safe range, he has more energy, feels better and thoroughly enjoys the reflexology effects.

I have worked on the feet of twenty-two persons (prayerfully applied). One, an autistic young woman, one man who is blind, one lovely ninety-four-year-old lady, and many others who all thank me graciously. I have people waiting for reflexology, including my minister.

A retired surgeon to whom I have been giving foot reflexology for almost two years tells me the pituitary gland alone is very important, and excretes valuable hormones into the blood. When he is in too much pain to sleep, he has his wife call me and he says I always ease his pain with my electric healing and reflex therapy.

It is wonderful, knowing how to relieve a headache . . . I was able to stop a terrible headache today in a blind man. He was left blind following a stroke which followed surgery. Recently his doctor told him that he needed prostate surgery. (He and his wife naturally did not consent to another surgery.) There I was with reflexology, and his wife says his symptoms have been relieved. I hope and pray he is all right.

I work hard giving reflexology to my family and friends, all with a lot of faith, hard work, and determination, and we're getting results. Thanks for reflexology and to our Heavenly Father. Thank you, I love you for what you are doing. You have taught me so much!

—P.C.

WORKING THE REFLEXES ON THE RIGHT FOOT

You have just stimulated all the reflex points on the left foot. Place both feet together and compare the difference in color. The left foot will have a healthy glow, while the right foot, which has not received much reflex attention as yet, will have a dull or diffused color. If you are in an area where there is a breeze or the air is cold, cover the left foot with a blanket, towel, or slipper.

Now you are ready to work the reflexes on the right foot. Remember that you have already warmed both feet up at the beginning of the session. Now you will want to begin reflexing the toes on this foot to stimulate the brain and nervous systems. These two systems control the body's movements and activities and relate to the functioning of all internal glands and organs.

Reflex the Toes First

Place the right foot into the same position as you had for the left one, holding it comfortably with your left or right hand, whichever is the more natural for you. Start with the big toe and press into the very center of the pad, feeling for the reflex to the hypothalamus, pituitary, and pineal reflexes; then check the whole toe for sore spots. The pain in the pituitary reflex is quite sharp, like a pin sticking into the toe, so work carefully at first. Work the entire big toe on the right foot and search out tender spots on all four sides and around the base of the toe, including the very tip.

Next proceed to work all the other toes, continuing the same course described for the left foot. (Remember the special spot that will stop many types of headache, on the inside of the second toe, just as it joins the foot.) This reflex point often releases a lot of tension in the neck area. Work on around the second toe, staying close to the big toe, and find another reflex point on top of the foot. This reflex corresponds to the upper lymph drainage in the neck area essential to healing.

Work all the other toes searching for sore spots and encouraging circulation to the head. Take one toe at a time between your fingers, work it and stretch it slightly. Then gently rotate it, first to the left, then to the right, about three times each way. Take your time and work all the reflexes as thoroughly as before, taking care to work all the toe reflexes on both feet equally well.

After you have worked all the reflex points on the toes, work on down to the reflexes of the throat, and then to the right eye and ear.

REFLEXING RIGHT SIDE OF THE THYROID

Use the right thumb to work the right foot, as you used the left thumb on the left foot. Walk your thumb just under the basal joint of the big toe in a pressing motion. Don't forget the parathyroid reflex is a bit deeper; however, it should receive adequate stimulation when you work the thyroid reflex.

If your reflex partner is having trouble with the thyroid, work around the big toe, including the top. Remember to also work the "assistant thyroid reflex" on the right foot if you did so on the left because it is important to work both feet equally.

HOW TO IMPROVE CIRCULATION TO THE SPINE

You should be familiar with the importance of the spine in the maintenance of the natural health of the body (refer to Chart H). Work the spine reflexes of the right foot in the same way that you worked those on the left foot.

Find the best position for working them, keeping in mind that the base of the toenail on the inside edge of the big toe is the beginning of the upper part of the spine. See the visual cross-section of spinal column reflexes in Chapter 7, pages 72 and 75.

Many times you can relax the spine enough, by working the reflexes, to enable it to go back into place by itself. But be aware that if it stays out of alignment, health problems will be persistent. If the spine reflexes continue to show a lot of tenderness after several sessions, recommend that your partner go to see a good chiropractor. It is not necessary for a chiropractor to use hard pressure to align the spine (which can actually be very harmful), so make sure you recommend someone who you know is careful and reputable.

Remember to stimulate the reflex area on top of the foot to benefit skeletal muscles, nerves, and blood vessels. Finger-walk from the spine, over the top of the foot toward the outside edge.

Work All Reflex Points on Both Feet

Of course you will want to work the reflex areas in the upper region of the right foot as thoroughly as you worked them in the left foot. We will not repeat the techniques here. So if you need to freshen your memory, just turn back a few pages to where you learned how to work the reflexes to the lung, thymus, adrenal, kidney, etc., on the left foot. The positions of holding the foot and the methods of working the reflex points will be the same except, of course, that you will be using the opposite foot and hands.

How to Stop Leg, Foot, or Toe Cramps

You may find that, while you are working the reflexes of another person, the toes, foot, or leg will go into a cramp. The first thing to do is have your reflex partner point the toes toward the nose; this straightens out the tendons and reduces the cramping in the lower legs. Then try rubbing the cords under the knee. If this doesn't help, then rub your hands together quickly and use the electric healing force from your own hands for a few minutes on the cramping area.

These cramps may recur several times during a reflex session, but will be less severe and will finally stop as the muscles become accustomed to the added circulation you are sending through them.

How to Tone the Liver With Reflexology

The liver, for all its size, is a very sensitive organ and is susceptible to damage from excessive alcohol, malnutrition, obesity, and various diseases. Read all you can about the liver. Once you have learned about this wonderful and vital organ, you will then take great care in working its reflex, knowing how many vital functions are dependent on it. The liver has an enormous amount of work to do and must perform at peak efficiency at all times if the rest of the body is to be kept in harmony and balance.

Working the Liver Reflex

To work the liver reflex, use the thumb of either hand. Start by holding the right foot in the right hand and placing the thumb of the left hand near the ball of the foot, under the little toe. With your thumb, begin pressing and working this area, searching for tender spots. The

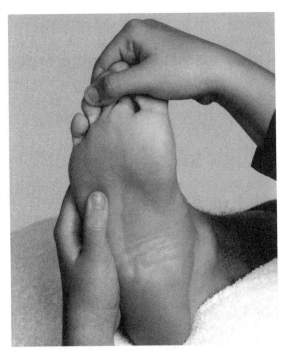

Photo 37. With right hand, slightly hold toes back to spread out reflex area. Use your left thumb to work across the large reflex area of the liver.

liver is a large gland, so you will need to reflex the whole area gently at first, increasing the pressure as you test the sensitivity of your partner's reflexes.

Criss-Cross Technique on the Liver Reflex

Since the liver does over 500 different things for the body and is amazingly versatile and regenerative, you will want to send energy currents to all its parts. One method especially beneficial to the liver is the criss-cross technique, which you used previously on the left foot. Work your thumb in a diagonal pattern from the waistline up toward the toes, using a slow press-and-roll motion. Change hands and work the other thumb in the same manner, crossing the paths of the first thumb. (See Illustration 15 on page 108.)

By criss-crossing this whole reflex area you may find hidden sore spots that you couldn't reach by reflexing one way. As is true of many of these reflexes, you will find them by changing hands and working from different angles. As reflexing becomes more natural to you, this method of searching out tender places will prove to be very effective and rewarding.

Keep in mind that the reflexes to a sluggish liver can be very painful and should be worked on with great caution the first few times. Whereas reflexes to other glands and organs may cause sharp, prickling sensations, those to a faulty liver will cause a dull ache which can be very painful to the reflex receiver.

The liver is one gland that can rebuild itself if given a chance. Nature has performed wisely here since the liver is so important. Don't overwork it during the first few sessions, as this could cause discomfort or illness. Use your own judgment in giving the liver adequate attention and encouraging the healing forces of regenerating or rebuilding.

STIMULATING THE GALLBLADDER AND DUODENUM

The gallbladder is attached to the underside of the liver. It is a pear-shaped sac which stores bile, or gall, from the liver, which is then squeezed out to help digest fats. Note on Chart B that the gallbladder will receive stimulation when the liver reflex is thoroughly worked. It is located a little on the lower edge of the liver on the right foot, comparable to the position of the spleen reflex on the left foot.

Try working the gallbladder at the lower edge of the liver reflex and work toward the center of the foot.

When there are gall stones you will have no trouble in locating the spot because you will find this area extremely sore. To reflex this you may have to use a very light feather touch at first, increasing the pressure as the pain subsides. Usually you will see much improvement after the first session. But the third session tells the story of improvement in almost all cases, not only for the reflexes to the liver but for all reflexes to all parts of the body.

The duodenum is the first ten inches of the small intestine. It receives bile and enzymes from the liver and pancreas, and plays a big part in the digestive system. It is more prominent on the right side. Its reflex is mostly in the soft tissue area of the right foot, akin to the stomach reflex on the left foot. This reflex is mostly stimulated as you work the reflexes to the liver, gallbladder, pancreas, and the transverse colon.

The stomach reflex on this foot should receive some attention. While the stomach lies mostly on the left side of the body, it is best to cover the reflexes on the right foot, too, because this "storage area" becomes stretched and often overlaps both sides of the body. Its reflex is found in the soft tissue area, just a little above the waistline of the foot.

The digestive tract contains a network of blood vessels which nourishes the stomach, and its nerves activate the muscles that move the food through the system. So, as you can see, you need to send vital energy to both sides of the mid torso by working the stomach reflex area in both feet, especially if there are signs of stomach trouble.

All My Life I Had Hoped for a Miracle

Dear Mrs. Carter and Tammy,

I hope this letter finds you in excellent health! I am writing you these few lines but I cannot find the right words to express how grateful and thankful I am to you. For twenty years I had suffered from pain on my right side. All my life I had hoped for a miracle and had gone from one doctor to another in Switzerland, Germany, Iran, Boston, and many in New York City. I was always diagnosed as having an ulcer or something. No one was able to help me, I was ready to go through an operation. Then I was lucky to get hold of your reflexology book. I tried reflexology, especially the reflexes to the liver and gallbladder and it helped my stomach, and intestines, etc. . . . Now I eat almost everything without any pain afterwards. My general health, vision, inner ear problems have improved so much. I went to the bookstore and purchased ten of each of your books. I sent them to my three sisters in Europe, my brother in Nevada, and other relatives.

I really believe in you and may God bless you for all of us. I can learn to help so many people in Europe and here in the USA who want help. I cannot thank you enough for all the good you have done for me and thank God for sending you to those of us who are willing to take care and heal illness the way nature meant it. Once again, thank you.

—N.G., New York

LOCATING THE ADRENAL AND KIDNEY REFLEX ON THE RIGHT FOOT

Right Adrenal Reflex . . . After you work the liver, move your hand down the foot just a bit to the adrenal reflex. Remember that this reflex is on top of the kidney reflex in the right foot, just as it is on the left foot. Use the same position for reflexing here, using, of course, the opposite hand. To refresh your memory of the physiology of the adrenals and kidneys, refer to Chapter 12.

Keep in mind that the reflex to the adrenal might be more sensitive on this foot than it was on the other, especially if the reflex to the pituitary and other endocrine glands showed sensitivity.

By remembering the tender spots, you will be able to double-check before you complete the session. Go back and press the area that was tender when you first reflexed it. See if it has improved any. Often you will find that much of the soreness has subsided. Sometimes there will still be the same tenderness, while other times the area may be completely free from any pain whatsoever.

Do not overwork the adrenal reflex since it is connected to the kidney, and you will not be able to work it without applying some pressure to the kidney reflex as well.

Right Kidney Reflex... You have learned the techniques of working the kidneys in Chapter 31. Also review Chapter 12. The right kidney reflex on the right foot should get the same workout as the left kidney reflex on the left foot. By now you know the exact procedure for working this reflex, using, of course, different hands. As stated previously, avoid overstimulation for the first few sessions.

WHERE TO LOCATE THE APPENDIX AND ILEOCECAL REFLEX

The ileocecal valve is where the small intestine connects to the colon. And almost in the same place, at the end of the colon, is a projecting pouch of skin, known as the vermiform appendix.

It may be hard to find these reflexes at first; refer to the illustration and to Chart B, and then test for soreness at the lower end of the ascending colon reflex. While holding the foot with the right hand, work with the thumb or knuckle of your left hand. This reflex will be just a little above the pad of the heel and toward the outside of the foot. Location of these reflexes may vary a little on different people, because weight and age will make a slight difference in how the colon is positioned.

The appendix is not essential to any known function. However, if it becomes diseased, it will become inflamed and can burst. If there is indication of an appendicitis attack, suggest strongly that the reflex receiver seek medical care. A ruptured appendix can be fatal if not attended to. Do not allow your reflex companion to have anything to eat or drink before going to the doctor. If there is old scar tissue from a previous appendectomy, this reflex may show tenderness but does not necessarily suggest that there is any current difficulty. When you are not sure, ask the reflex receiver about any previous trouble in this area.

You may have to use a tool to get in deep enough on this reflex, especially if it is on a receiver whose feet have an extra thick sole. It will often be impossible to reflex deeply enough to do much good with the fingers alone. When you press in the general area of the appendix or ileocecal valve with a test-and-hunt method, your partner will let you know when you have found the right spot if there is any

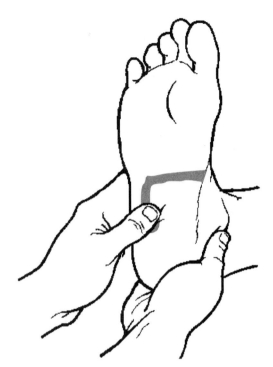

Illustration 37. Position for working the reflex to the appendix and ileo-cecal valve which is located on the right foot.

congestion in the area at all. With a little experience you will be able to pinpoint the reflexes on the first try.

How to Activate the Ascending and Transverse Colon

The colon, of course, is part of the gastrointestinal system and is approximately six feet long. Its reflex is quite lengthy and crosses over both feet. In Chapter 32, you learned how to stimulate the left half of the colon on the left foot; now you will reflex the right foot. Notice that each time the colon makes a turn it has a different "name" to help us identify which part of the colon we are referring to; however, it is all one large intestine.

The manner of working this reflex on the right foot will differ from that on the left foot. Instead of starting in the middle of the foot near the spine reflex, you will start on the outside pad of the heel, between the fourth and fifth zones. Work up toward the waistline of the foot with the pressing-rolling motion. When you get to the waistline of the foot, change the position of your left hand and work across the foot, toward the spine reflex area, with the same press-and-roll motion. If there is trouble here, work the path of this reflex many times. Continue to cover the whole colon area often, checking for special sore spots which will indicate that there is congestion in the bowel. Keep in mind that the colon reflexes can be very painful in some people. So start out gently, increasing the pressure as the tenderness subsides.

You recall that in Chapter 32, page 267, you learned to crisscross the whole lower torso area for troubles of constipation or colon toxicity. If you worked the left foot for these conditions, remember to also work the right foot in the same way, diagonally from the waistline down to the heel, reverse directions, and work back up the heel.

Healthy bowel and colon function is very important to everyone. If someone has symptoms of infrequent bowel movements, constant bad breath, headaches, or excessive gas, recommend improving the diet, a plan of exercise, and the advantages of reflexology.

REVIEWING REFLEXES OF THE LOWER REGION

Study the charts and become completely familiar with all reflexes on both feet. Learn which are the same on both feet; the intestine and bladder reflexes are good examples. You will not be given repetitive full directions for the right foot, as the techniques are the same as those you have already learned in earlier chapters. You will, of course, use the opposite hands when working the right foot. Never neglect to give both feet the same amount of reflexing, because you must send a balanced force of vital life energy surging along specific pathways to bring renewed life and healing to the *whole* body.

Here we will recap the reflex locations explained earlier. As you retrace the reflex stimulation points on the right foot, remember to give each reflex area your full attention.

Recalling How to Work the Reflexes for Intestines

Continue using the same reflex methods to the intestines on the right foot as you did on the left foot. If you are not completely familiar with the procedure, re-read pages 265–267. Use the opposite hands, of course, when working the right foot.

Highlighting the Bladder, Lower Lumbar, and Reflexes to Help Hemorrhoid Problems

The Bladder . . . another organ that you have already learned to reflex. Now use the same technique here on the right foot as you used on the left, changing hands, of course.

The Lower Lumbar . . . Reflex the lower lumbar area (which is the lower vertebraes and end of the spine, in the same way as you did on the left foot. This section of the vertebrae is significantly larger than the rest of the spine. Nature made it this way because it supports most of the upper body weight.

You recall that the bladder reflex is in the same location. However, the reflex to the lumbar area is slightly deeper and closer to the ankle and heel, so you will need to press on past the bladder reflex to reach the reflex of the lower lumbar. Reflexing this area will also help relieve pain in other parts of the lower extremities such as the sciatic nerve, prostate trouble, and female disorders. Getting circulation to this area can also help to relieve lower backaches.

Hemorrhoids . . . You have acquired the information from your charts, and from working on the left foot, that there are reflex areas around the heels and up the cord on back of the leg to relieve the pain of hemorrhoids. The bladder and lower lumbar reflex location is also very close to the rectum reflex, and is often effective as an assistant reflex.

Straining because of constipation can cause veins and capillaries to swell, thereby bringing on the discomfort of hemorrhoids. Stimulation to the rectum reflex helps promote renewed circulation within this zone.

Remembering How to Reflex the Sciatic Nerve, Hip/Shoulder, and Reproductive Glands

Sciatic Nerve . . . You learned from a complete coverage in Chapter 32 how to reflex the areas of the sciatic nerve. So now you should be familiar with the technique involved. Another assistant helper for sciatic pain is the hip reflex on the outside of the foot (see Illustration 36 on page 288).

Hip/Shoulder . . . Work the outer edge of the foot, using thumb-walk or the criss-cross technique. If your thumbs are becoming fatigued, you may want to use your index and middle finger to work this area.

Reproductive Glands . . . Remember how nature placed the reflexes to these delicate organs and glands in a protected area, up on the sides of the feet, under the ankles. Keep in mind that the penis, prostate and uterus are not located on one side of the body or the other, but are in the center, and each consists of one organ only. Do not forget to give these important reflexes equal attention on both feet.

Strengthening the Immune System

Lymph . . . Be sure all lymph reflexes are well covered in every reflex session you give, since they take care of all infections and help protect the body from disease. You may need to refer to your "mental notes" to recollect if earlier in the session any of the larger lymph node reflexes you covered were sore. (These would be the thymus, spleen, and tonsils.) If they showed signs of tenderness, give this reflex area some extra attention so that its circulation will be improved enough to filter out any disease-causing organisms.

Note: When referring to the techniques used in photos or illustrations for the left foot, remember now that you have changed feet for reflexing, so you must alternate hands. Always keep the reflex-receiver comfortable and use whatever procedure you find least fatiguing. Follow the proper routine for working each reflex, and take as much time as necessary for a thorough and beneficial reflexology session.

Conclude the Session With Your Favorite Relaxing Technique

You have given a complete reflex session, and have thoroughly worked all the reflexes of both feet. Now finish the workout with one or more of the following techniques: the foot-and-ankle shuttle, the solar-plexus-press, or a few slow and relaxing foot and toe rotations. Any one, or all, of these routines can be beneficial. Be aware that tension is the cause of many illnesses, and relaxing your reflex partner with reflexology is helping the powers of nature in the wonderful work of healing.

Ease Body Stress with the Foot-and-Ankle Shuttle

Place one hand on the lateral and one on the medial side of the foot, where the basal joints of the toes join the foot. Use slight pressure with each hand, gently rolling the foot back and forth between your hands. Move hands to the ankle area of the foot, and repeat the push-and-pull motion with your hands. (Refer to Illustrations 19a, 19b and 19c, pages 222-223.) This routine is very comforting to the receiver.

Calm Nervous Tensions with the Solar-Plexus-Press

Place both thumbs on the solar plexus reflex buttons on both feet at the same time. This reflex is in the center of the arch just below the ball of the foot, at the diaphragm region. After some practice, your fingers will fall automatically into place on each reflex point as you come to it. With your thumbs positioned into the solar plexus reflex

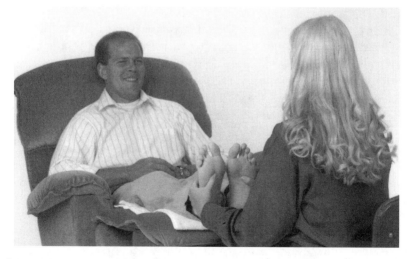

Photo 38. Use the solar-plexus-press on both feet simultaneously. This double-thumb reflex technique is rewarding to the whole body.

in the center of each foot, ask your partner to slowly breathe air into the lungs. As a deep breath is taken, gradually push your thumbs into the feet, hold for ten seconds, then slowly release the pressure as your partner also slowly releases the breath. (You can breathe along with your partner if you like.) Repeat two or three times at first. This may take a little practice, but is well worth it, as it is a very relaxing and rewarding process.

Relax the Mind and Body with Foot and Toe Rotations

Take one foot and rotate it, first to the left, then to the right. Repeat on the other foot. This is very relaxing for the whole system.

Now rotate each toe, then end with a slight, gentle pull; do this to all ten toes to stimulate circulation. You may end the session with an electric massage of each foot for a few seconds if you wish. Let your companion rest for a while if need be, as the anatomy's own healing powers work best while the body is totally relaxed.

Refresh Yourself

To disperse negative vibrations or tired muscles, shake your hands at your sides about six times (as if shaking water from your fingertips). Wash hands with cold running water to dispel any accumulated hand or finger fatigue.

If the feet you just worked on had any type of unfriendly bacteria, wash with soap and rinse with a disinfectant or rubbing alcohol. After drying your hands, apply a refreshing hand cream. Moisturizers with aloe vera and vitamin E are not oily, and can be used during the day or at night to protect your skin. This way your hands will be clean, soft, and smooth for giving another healthful reflex workout to someone who needs your comforting touch.

REFLEXOLOGY BENEFITS MANY

Reflexology is a natural way to help safeguard health. It helps to induce tranquil relaxation. It aids nature in cleansing the body of harmful impurities; it balances and revitalizes the whole body. We hear this not only from reflexology professionals but from the general public as well who have helped themselves and others with overwhelming success. Following are a few testimonies from some who have uplifted their families and friends with reflexology's wonderful healing powers.

Dear Mrs. Carter,

I have been using reflexology on my daughter whom I wrote to you about some time ago. It has done wonders for her. I have helped many friends to help themselves. Your help should be known throughout the whole world. It is doing what doctors have failed to do. Thank you for your help and may God give you wisdom and knowledge to fight on for mankind.

Best Wishes,
—E.L.

Reflexology Has Changed My Life

Dear Mrs. Carter,

Your book *Helping Yourself with Foot Reflexology* has changed my life. Would you believe that I cured myself of eyesight trouble? I have been wearing glasses for the past 20 years. I have been studying your books for seven years now, and they have given me great satisfaction, both for myself and to watch others recuperate under my very eyes in just a short time. Since I was a child, I have loved to help the sick and the weary, and have prayed to God to open a door for me, so that I could help people naturally, something beyond medical aid.

Late one night, a young boy woke me up, telling me his father had a lot of pain in his leg. I went to the father and found this to be true. I told him I did not have any medicine, but that I knew of something far better. While I was checking his leg, I noticed a swollen portion which was turning blue. The nearest doctor was sixty miles from us, and it was in the middle of the night. I knew this could be a blood clot or congestion in his leg through tension. I had to do my best in this situation. I used rubber bands on his toes to stop the pain within the zone. Then used reflexology on the whole foot to stimulate circulation. What a miracle; within three minutes the pain was gone and the swelling was going away. God bless you for this wonderful research to enable us to help people in seconds!

Sincerely,
—C.L.B.,
Secunda, S.A.

Nature's Healing Powers, Better than "Pain Pill"

Dear Mrs. Carter,

Nature is the healer of my body. Nature's healing powers are much more effective than any "pain pill" made by men, and doesn't cost a dime! I have had several aches and pains in my back and neck over the years and always I would take an aspirin to relieve the pain, but now I am brought instant relief by working the corresponding spine and neck reflex areas found in my feet.

My dad is 61 years old and just retired last year. He often complained about the pains and cramps in his legs. I have helped him a great deal by working the sciatic nerve reflexes that you showed me, and now he very seldom complains about his legs; but when he does, I grab a foot. I wish you could have seen my mom and dad before I started using reflexology on them, so you could see how much they have improved. Thank you for showing me this wonderful technique.

—Mr. E.C.
Texas

CHAPTER 35

Reflexology Knowledge Is the Sign of Wisdom

From the beginning of time, the human body has been a never-ending source of wonderment to its owner. Through the knowledge of reflexology you will also gain an understanding about the body's structure and how it functions. Your reflexology education will lead to an increased appreciation of how the body is organized; each gland and organ tirelessly does its own job, and yet no one part of the body is designed to function alone. The more you experience the accomplishments of reflexology, the more aware you will become of your body's beauty and wonder.

Much scientific research is taking place, with studies that demonstrate the effectiveness of reflexology, and how its use is helping hundreds of people achieve optimum health. Reflexology associations around the world are reporting wonderful case studies of how professional reflexologists are working in hospitals, physical therapy centers, and crisis clinics. These reports verify a high percentage of improved results with their clients.

REFLEXOLOGY GIVES NATURE A HELPING HAND

Reflexology is a natural method of healing that focuses on helping the body take care of its own needs. One of the main principles of good health is to keep the circulation moving to prevent accumulated waste materials from building up in the body over a period of time. The body is self-initiated to throw off naturally any waste or toxic accumulations that may be interfering with its proper functioning.

Reflexology will stimulate this renewed circulation to help the body flush out these unwanted materials and help it return to its original healthy condition. Many have learned that by using reflexology the body can obtain proper balance, recover from illness, and regenerate new cells for a healthy new lifestyle.

Everywhere we go we hear how not only the general public, but the conventional medical profession as well, is becoming more and more interested in its natural healing process. Doctors and pharmaceutics are starting to recognize the fact that surgery and drugs are not always the best practicable care for their patients. It is good news that both doctors and scientists are becoming open-minded and are taking a closer look at various methods of natural healing. Moreover, valued research and special surveys indicate an increasing number of individuals who are beginning to recognize the desirability of learning how to use the healing forces of nature to bring relief, and in many cases, complete and permanent healings by the simple technique of working the reflex points. Let us enlighten you with the following case studies.

FOOT REFLEXOLOGY AND DIABETES

This interesting study was printed in the *Foot Reflexology Awareness Association News Report*:

Thirty-two cases of Type II diabetes mellitus were randomly divided into two groups. One group was treated with *conventional Western medicine and foot reflexology*, the other with the same *medicine but without any reflexology*. After 30 days of treatment, blood glucose levels, platelet aggregation, length and net weight of the thrombus, senility symptom scores and serum lipid perodide were *"greatly reduced" in the foot reflexology group* . . . while *"no significant change" was observed in the group that took its medicine without any reflexology*. This study signified that foot reflexology was an effective treatment for Type II diabetes mellitus.

"Treating Type II diabetes mellitus with foot reflexotherapy," Wang, XM; First Teaching Hospital, Beijing Medical University, China, 1993.

THE IMPORTANCE OF WORKING
THE CORRECT REFLEX POINTS

Terry Oleson, Ph.D., and William Flocco, Director of the American Academy of Reflexology, conducted a randomized, controlled study of premenstrual symptoms involving stimulation of reflex points on the ears, hands, and feet. Results of their clinical findings were published in the December 1993 issue of the major medical journal *Obstetrics & Gynecology.*

Their objective was to determine whether "true reflexology techniques" would reduce PMS distress more effectively than using "false reflexology techniques." After carefully interviewing many women who reported premenstrual symptoms, they chose thirty-five individuals who had never experienced extensive prior reflexology. None of them was pregnant; none was taking estrogen or progesterone specifically for PMS.

The women were divided into two groups. Each received a thirty-minute reflexology session once a week, given to them by a trained reflexology therapist. *One group received 100% correct* and appropriate reflexology treatments on their ears, hands, and feet. The reflex points that were stimulated *did* correspond to specific areas of the body that *do* relate to PMS problems. The appropriate reflexes were to such areas as the uterus, ovaries, endocrine system, etc. *The other half received a placebo,* which was inappropriate reflex treatments on their ears, hands, and feet. The reflex points that were stimulated *did not* correspond to any specific areas of the body that related to PMS problems. Instead the therapists worked on reflex areas that corresponded to the shoulder, upper arm, elbow, etc., which did encourage some circulation; however, not to the correct zones. Since none of these women were familiar with reflexology pressure points or procedures, no one knew which group she was in. However, each participant found that reflexology was relaxing and pleasant.

Each woman kept a daily diary for six months: two months before the reflex sessions started, two months during reflex treatments, and two months afterward. She would record somatic and psychological distresses and monitor 38 premenstrual symptoms. The volunteers in the study showed similar charting of PMS symptoms before the treatment period started.

Results indicated that women who received genuine reflex therapy, corresponding to correct regions of the body, showed a 46 percent reduction in premenstrual symptoms. This was a much greater reduction than the 19 percent reduction of those who received the placebo reflex pressure which had very little therapeutic value for those who suffer PMS.

There was a remarkable difference between how the two groups felt, even in the two months after this experimental study had been completed. Those who received 100% truthful reflexology had a much greater reduction in their PMS discomforts. The results of this study prove that reflexology to the *correct reflex points* makes a significant difference!

REFLEXOLOGY IS THE NATURAL WAY TO BETTER HEALTH

Reflexology is known as an alternative/complementary medicine in many countries around the world where it is generally practiced. For example, it is used in Israeli hospitals where they are covered by national health care insurance. In Great Britain qualified reflexology practitioners promote good health and natural healing and proudly provide continuing education and training to benefit the public. These reflexologists are helping out wherever they are needed, such as with HIV-positive clients. Reflex therapists do not offer a cure of the condition, yet they know that in a person's darkest hour, there is immense comfort and nourishment from the therapeutic touch of caring hands.

A case study from London is a wonderful testimony of how one reflexologist worked with a doctor, therapist, and family to help a young victim of brain damage return to a normal life.

We hear also about adventurous people like Father Joseph who brings his valuable curative reflexology methods to several areas of Asia, helping those who cannot afford medical care. He is praised for his efforts to help stop pain and prevent disease. He teaches individuals about the benefits of reflexology, and advises them to reject activities harmful to their health.

Reflexologists everywhere are highly respected, and they are the people who will make a difference in the world, promoting renewed health and doing what they can to preserve the world's greatest wonder . . . human life. Following are a few notes from readers who have benefited from reflexology.

Dear Mrs. Carter,

I have read, studied and applied the treatments taught in your books, Mildred Carter! I have been able to help many people for the past fourteen years with great success in Florida, Canada, California and now in Mexico, where I have lived for the past two and one-half years.

I live on a sailing vessel, and have for the past sixteen years. My child was born and I have used reflexology on him from the age of three until now (he is fourteen). He has never had any children's diseases, has never seen a doctor, and never wants to see one!

I have been able to help many sailor friends and recommend your books to all! The NEED IS GREAT for natural health care here in Mexico on the out-islands. A lot of work has to be done, and the Mexicans love it! Willingly they will give you their feet and hands and will learn to do reflexology on themselves. Thanks to your wonderful teachings, which I appreciate enormously.

—M.E., Mexico

Dear Mrs. Carter,

Reflexology is WONDERFUL, truly a blessing from God. You, dear Mildred Carter, are an instrument of God. I have had rheumatoid arthritis since I was 35 years old; now I am just fine. Have been telling everyone about your work. I am now 63 years of age and feel like a young child, thanks to God and your wonderful books. God bless you always, dear lady.

Sincerely,
—J.M.

Dear Mrs. Carter,

I am seventy-two years, and retired. I have arthritis in my knees. There are a lot of people in this area who have "bad" knees and a lot have "new joints" put in, or operated on. Some of us went to a reflexologist here in town. She helped more than the doctor or chiropractor. My wife is learning all that she can too. In this way we can help out one another, our friends and relatives.

—J.H.

Dear Mrs. Carter and Mrs. Weber,

After learning the proper method of reflexology, I will be able to relieve people from their pain and illness with the help of nature. Reflexology is a way to health naturally without drugs. It will be something I can use for the rest of my life to make the world a safer, healthier, happier place to live in.

—S.B., Wisconsin

Dear Mrs. Carter,

Recently I had the opportunity to look at a copy of your book *Body Reflexology*. Thank you for the wealth of information it contains. You obviously have done a great deal of research. I have been reading books about iridology, reflexology, etc., for a number of years now. I was impressed by the comprehensive and easy-to-follow style of your book. It is written in such a way that I found myself eager to try some of the things you suggested. The immediate results obtained were a pleasant surprise.

I was most interested in the "Formula for a Sick Colon" on page 147. I know that chlorophyll plays an important part in a healthy colon because mine shuts down and refuses to work at all without it. May God bless you as you continue to use and share His natural healing methods.

Cordially yours,
—M.F., Texas

"While walking, my husband was hit by a car and put through a windshield. While he was in a coma for months, I used reflexology to bring the brain around and to bring feeling into the body. As of today, he is trying to say words and do things the doctors said he would never do, and I feel it is from me working on his feet when it was needed."

Thank you,
—J.N.

"It is amazing to me how marvelously made the body is. I have always avoided medication unless absolutely necessary and have been conscientious about good nutrition. Now, this discovery of how to overtly aid the body in the process of detoxification, elimination and healing is the perfect correlation to good nutrition."

"For years I have been aware of the role the endocrine system plays in maintaining health of the body, but I was never aware of the fact that you could stimulate it (in a good way) and bring it back to a normal working state. I find it exciting and rewarding to be able to use reflexology, and reflex away someone's headache, or depression, or fatigue. I am really looking forward to learning more."

—C.E.
Texas

"Thank you for your most wonderful books on reflexology which have been of great help to me. I have also studied Touch for Health techniques, which link very closely with reflexology. We can't do enough to take responsibility for our own health. Rejuvenation techniques are of particular interest to me. Natural therapies are gaining increasing acceptance here in Australia . . . good news indeed!"

With thanks! Yours sincerely,
—N.L.
Australia

"I use your hand and foot reflexology books, and also my Foot-Reflexology-Roller every night and morning. I will be 82 on Monday and people say I look like I am in my

60's . . . and I feel GOOD, and I am active. I believe it could be my reflexology that is the main reason for my youthfulness, and of course vitamins and minerals too."

Thank you,
—O.L.

"I am not usually an affluent letter writer but I do want you to know that your books have been a GREAT blessing to me and mine for quite some years, and have saved us MANY dollars in doctor bills, with great relief from pain and misery.

Thank you so much for your labor of love and sharing with us. God bless and reward you abundantly."

Most sincerely yours,
—A.M.
Washington

"I have had a spur on my spine. Six years ago the spur looked like a fish hook. Ultrasound is what they have used on me. I wanted you to know by using the spine reflexes on my feet, it reduced the pain in my back considerably. God made the body perfect, never to grow old. No wonder the body can heal itself. I don't believe our bodies need all these painkillers. Reflexology is the answer."

—M.B.

"My thirteen stays in local hospitals amounted to over $65,000 and I was still struggling. In just a few days of using reflexology, my asthma has diminished and I feel renewed energy. Thank you for your wonderful book and caring."

—P.H.

"It is most inspiring to know that by the simple technique of reflexology we can do so much to help our fellow man. It is simple but, oh so powerful once we learn how to use it correctly for the good of all. To me it is perhaps one of the greatest tools or means of relieving much suffering, yet without using harmful substances or damaging the structure of the body temple."

—G.G.
Texas

"I am so glad I started reading your books. You are the greatest for sharing so much with so many. Your teachings work for the fastest, greatest results I have ever witnessed!"

Thank you so much!
—S.J.C.

"I have purchased every one of your books, and never dreamed anything as wonderful as reflexology could be so easy to help the ailing body. I had first read your book *Helping Yourself with Foot Reflexology* about four years ago. I call it MY MAGIC HEALER. I have helped my friends and family, including myself, so many times. I can't thank you enough; you truly are a God-Send Person to be so much help to so many people in the world with your wonderful books. I am really ready to help the people I love, with your wonderful way of healing."

God bless you,
—Mr. D.Y.

"I must tell you that what you have done to free up the people from pain and suffering is one of the greatest things for humanity. And every child in school should have a class to study and learn reflexology!"

Fondly,
—R.B.
Nevada

"I always have stomach upsets at work after eating lunch. Now that I have learned how to work the reflexes to the stomach, the upset is gone. It really works for me!"

—M.B.

"I have had your book for about a year. Reflexology shows me how you do not have to fill your body with a lot of poison to be free from pain.

The medical profession gave up on me as a patient because doctors did not know what to do for me. I could not live a normal life for having muscle spasms all over my body. A friend told me about a reflexologist so I tried her. Now I am leading a normal life. I am so happy to learn reflexology, so I can help others like I have been helped. I am so excited with this knowledge, I tell everyone I meet. Thanks!"

Yours truly,
—E.C., Mississippi

TAKING CARE OF YOUR FEET

Using reflexology will help you focus more on the health of your feet; when they feel good, you feel good. Feet are our structural foundation, and are essential to our daily work, our physical activities, and the functioning of the entire body.

Always make sure your shoes fit your feet, without putting pressure on the toes. Your shoes should always have ample room for your toes so that you do not get corns or calluses. Some people say that when their feet hurt, they hurt all over. Anecdotal history has it that Abraham Lincoln had very large feet (size 14B shoe) and suffered with chronic, gnawing pain for which he had a private foot doctor who cared for his feet on a regular basis. He was quoted as often saying, "I cannot think if my feet hurt me!"

Survey Proves Feet Need Stimulation

Research was conducted a few years ago to see if wearing shoes had anything to do with foot problems. The survey was taken in India and

China with natives who habitually went barefoot, and was compared with a survey taken in the United States with people who wore shoes everyday. It showed that 85 percent of 5,000 surveyed adults in the U.S. had foot defects. On the other hand, in the India-China survey, only 7 percent of the 5,000 natives studied had any foot defects.

This illustrates the importance of nature's natural method of going barefoot. Of course this is not always possible, so, if we must wear shoes, we must also take time for reflexology! The stimulation will not only contribute to our healthful living, but it will also be pleasurable to our feet. And when we make our feet happy, they will make us happy!

Reflexology Helps Dissolve Spurs

Dear Mrs. Carter,

At first I was rather reluctant to try my hand at reflexology, but remembering back about ten years, when I had bad trouble with my feet and was about to have surgery on my heels for spurs, I changed my mind and went to see a foot reflexologist. My first visit was very painful and I had doubts about going back to her for treatment, but I did. After three or four more treatments, my heels no longer hurt, and ten years later they are still okay . . . No more pain in my heels!

My daughter also received treatment from her for a "stomach disorder" and was okay after only ONE visit.

—B.G.

REFLEXOLOGY IS AN EXTENSION TO OTHER HEALTH CARE PROGRAMS

Reflexology is used in many countries as a prescription for preventive health care. However, doing reflexology does not make you a qualified doctor, and if you have a friend who obviously needs the guidance of a health care professional, you can suggest seeking medical care. Reflexology is not intended to replace ongoing medical treatment.

When giving someone else reflexology, your role is not actually to diagnose merely to bring relief. But if a person has waited too long to turn to nature's own method through reflexology, he or she may need the immediate attention of a conscientious doctor. You as a reflexologist are an ally of the medical profession, and must not say things to make others lose faith in it. Reflexology is an extension of other health care programs when they are needed, and is not a substitute for needed medical or emergency care. Here is a list of ten emergency situations that we feel deserve to be mentioned.

When to Call a Medical Doctor

1. As a general rule, if you are concerned about the severity of a condition, or if there is a situation that you don't know how to handle, and there seems to be a great deal of pain involved, it is best to call a doctor. Some situations demand the immediate care of a physician, so by all means, seek medical help in these circumstances.

2. You should take someone to the hospital or call an ambulance in case of emergencies such as bone fractures, severe burns, hemorrhaging (bleeding from coughing up blood or bleeding from the urinary tract or rectum). Follow the same procedure if bleeding does not subside from a wound or nosebleed, especially in small children, as extensive loss of blood can lead to shock.

3. Convulsions or poisoning can also be cause for alarm. Accidental chemical poisoning is fatal if not treated in time. Adults and children who live in the country should learn what plants and berries are hazardous or poisonous. Also dangerous is poison from a rabied animal, or from a poisonous snake, or spider bite.

4. It is good to know CPR (cardiopulmonary resuscitation) which could be life-saving in an emergency if a person's heart and breathing have stopped. (Without the flow of blood through the heart, brain damage will occur.) This could happen in the case of a sunstroke, a heart attack or when someone who can't breathe is unconscious and/or turning blue. Even if you know first aid, call out for someone to dial 911 while you assist with CPR.

5. If there is a serious accident with an automobile, motorcycle or other type of mishap, waste no time, call for medical care immediately.

6. Proper diagnosis from a medical doctor is essential in some situations. For instance, life-saving surgery is essential for a ruptured appendix; certain medications may be needed for severe bacterial infections, or to avoid heart attacks or other disorders.

7. It's time to see a doctor if there is persistent vomiting or diarrhea, because the body loses fluids and electrolytes (body chemicals) which may cause severe dehydration and even shock.

8. If someone you know all of a sudden cannot talk or has slurred speech, or if a person gets dizzy and cannot see what is close by, that person should be checked by a physician, because these could be signs of a stroke.

9. Any time there are extreme chest pains or abrupt and severe abdominal pains, a doctor should be consulted.

10. If you work, travel, or live with someone who is on medication for mental disorders, diabetes, heart problems, epilepsy, or any other serious medical condition, you must find out how much medication to give if a difficulty should arise. Be prepared.

Read a guide to first aid for advice on family care, and if you have small children or grandchildren, learn how to prevent accidents and poisonings. Learning about such things as choking, drowning, etc., will help prepare you if an emergency were to arise when you would have to know what action to take. You will need to use your own judgment and intuition, so be ready to act quickly if an emergency was ever to happen near you.

How Mental Health Can Be Improved with Reflexology

As we have seen in this book, the body is not merely a machine which gets out of order here and there, but a delicately balanced system which must function smoothly and efficiently. The degree of its efficiency seems to have a direct connection with one's mental health. Conversely, a state of worry, tension, or anxiety can affect various organs and glands and bring on distressing physical ailments. So dependent and inseparable are the two aspects of man—mental and physical—that many cases of nervousness, indigestion, premature senility, irritability, depression, and even some cases of mental retardation, have their origin in a malfunctioning body.

Reflexology is Nature's own method of restoring the body to full efficiency, which in turn has a beneficial effect on the personality as tensions give way to peace of mind.

THE RULE OF RELAXATION FOR MENTAL HEALTH

The first rule for regaining peace of mind is relaxation, but one cannot relax when the body is shouting protests, and how can a person radiate love and harmony if the mind is in a turmoil? The most common remedy for physical or mental distress is to put something in the mouth instead of attacking the source, and relief always seems to be just around the corner in the next drugstore.

Now we all know that there is no miracle pill that can really relieve the body of strain or the mind of stress, except temporarily. Our environment has become so complicated that many people live in a state of fear and are willing to try almost anything for escape. Some turn to sedatives or alcohol, some find refuge in cigarettes, watching fights, gambling—whatever diverts the attention momentarily. Some take up causes, or sex, or war, or join unhealthy affiliations. A few are driven to that final resort, suicide. Still, the problem is not solved, and will remain unresolved until the person turns within to find the answers. To be able to relax for quiet meditation, one must be relaxed not only in mind but in body as well.

In this push-button age, we have overlooked Nature's own push buttons, right in the bottom of the feet. All you have to do is push them or walk them on a rough surface. What could be simpler and more rewarding than this simple but powerful push-button method which takes care of the body and the mind at the same time?

REFLEXOLOGY FOR MENTAL BENEFITS

Those who turn to reflexology, nature's own marvelous invention, will come closest to discovering the freedom for which they are searching. With renewed joy and youthful vigor, the disposition improves, efficiency increases, tasks are approached with eagerness and not apprehension, and the whole personality radiates love and optimism.

The vibrations that you send up to the pituitary gland with reflexology are filled with a power that will blend the whole system into harmony—and all you have to do is press the reflex button in the center of your big toe to start the vibrations of health swinging into action. The hypothalamus regulates pituitary secretions, and the pituitary gland controls the activity in all the other glands. It is no wonder that the hypothalamus and pituitary gland are called the "king glands"!

Then, as you proceed to work the other reflexes, you will feel an immediate response as the process of eliminating poisons from your systems commences. Remember that you are awakening sluggish glands and freeing them from the congestions that are affecting your very life. For this reason, you must remember not to be overeager for faster results by overdoing the reflex therapy at first. Start the treatment gently for a few seconds, then wait two or three days before you reflex again. This will give the body time to readjust itself. Just as a champion runner must train the muscles gradually, the body is in no condition to assume full efficiency without time.

HOW REFLEXOLOGY CAN IMPROVE EVERYONE'S CHARACTER

Life certainly does present its challenges: Dealing with a nerve-wracking job, the monotonous grind of household chores, pressure of schedules, the daily "rat-race" of earning a living, trying to keep up with the times which means buy-buy-buy, bigger bills, and higher taxes, commuting, shopping, child care, activities. The vitality wanes, there are symptoms of mental fatigue, and we become cross, irritable, and unpleasant.

Reflexology Break vs. Coffee Break

There is no need to allow such a mental condition to develop. Instead of a "coffee break" or a dose of sedatives, take a reflexology break and see how quickly you feel a recharge of vitality rushing through you. The reflex buttons in the bottoms of your feet are there as a gift from Nature to give you an energy boost any time you need it. All you have to do is sit down for five minutes and reflex them for a fast pick-up, and you will receive as an extra bonus, a wonderful feeling of well-being.

How to Improve Your Disposition

Do you realize that if every gland and organ in your body were in complete harmony with the universe and functioning properly, you would not let even the big things get you down, let alone life's minor irritations?

No one can have a sunny disposition if he or she is feeling under par. Tension from fear and worry can and does throw the body out of chemical balance. It tends to weaken the whole human organism, *especially the adrenal glands*, and if the supply of adrenal hormones runs dry, it can lead to various crippling diseases. Even though there is no sudden attack of illness of any kind, the body has actually been under a period of deterioration possibly for many years. A relaxed mind leads to relaxed nerves, and relaxed nerves make for a healthy body and a pleasant disposition.

"But how can I get rid of my worries and tensions?" you ask. *It is so simple, once you know the secrets of reflexology.* You can press a few reflex-buttons while relaxing in front of the TV and regain all the pep and vigor of your youth.

Why not use this marvelous method of rejuvenation to catapult yourself into a new way of life and become the true person you were meant to be, and that your family or friends certainly want you to be? Instead of a coffee break or a beer break, try a reflexology break first and enjoy every day to its very fullest for the rest of your life. This book shows you the way to do it.

Nature's Way to Control Stress

Reflexology is nature's helper, and what a wonder it is! Research indicates that when the body is stressed, it is more susceptible to disease. Reflex therapy is a safe, simple, and effective means to relieve stress and dissolve tension all over the body. When mental and physical tensions are reduced, the blood supply improves and promotes better circulation and nerve functioning. Soon the whole body is able to reestablish harmony within, obtain proper balance, and allow all systems to normalize themselves. As tension gives way to relaxation, the mind soon becomes peaceful and calm, which then gives nature the opportunity to restore and renew the body. It is truly one of nature's natural wonders, and a key to perfect health!

EXTREME MENTAL CASES HELPED

During my years of treating people with reflexology, I have come across many cases of mental stress—some of them minor and some so serious as to require commitment to an asylum. A colleague told me of cases which she had treated who were patients, some so agitated that they had become dangerous. With reflexology, she had been able to restore some of them to the point where they could return home.

How a Mentally Confused Teacher Was Helped

I remember one case of mine, a man whose family did not want to have committed. His wife asked me to come to the house to see if reflexology could be of any help.

"We don't really think that just rubbing the feet will do much good, but we are willing to try anything," she pleaded.

When I arrived, Mrs. D. met me at the door, her eyes filled with fear and exhaustion. Mr. D. was still a young man, and had been teaching school. He had become increasingly nervous and irritable the past few months, and the school was finally forced to ask him to take a leave of absence. Now he was having spells of violence and didn't seem to know what he was doing. The doctor prescribed sedatives, but he refused to take them. The wife had become so afraid of him that she had sent the children to stay with her mother.

"I'm afraid to let you go in," said Mrs. D. as she led me to the bedroom.

"Now, you leave me alone with him, and don't worry," I said. "I will be able to handle him, and I'll have him like a lamb in no time!" I could see a faint glimmer of hope light up in her eyes as I went into the room and closed the door.

The room was a mess, and so was Mr. D. He needed a haircut and a shave. His bedding was scattered on the floor, and he had torn his night clothes to shreds. He looked as if he had reverted to an animal. His eyes were wild as if he were trapped and ready to spring at me at any moment.

I felt a deep pity for this poor, mentally disturbed man, but no fear as I talked gently to him, telling him that I had come to rub his feet and relieve his tensions. I kept repeating that rubbing his feet would make him feel relaxed and help him to sleep. He watched me, wild-eyed, as I slowly approached the bed where he crouched ready to bolt and run. He didn't move, however, as I sat on the edge of the bed. I carefully took one of his feet in my hands, and began rubbing it very gently. He began to relax a little.

As soon as I felt that he was ready to trust me, I explained what I was going to do to his feet, and that it might hurt a little but that this was necessary to help him get well. He seemed to be listening intently, although his eyes still looked wild and untrusting.

Ever so lightly, I pressed on the reflex to the pituitary in the center of the big toe. As expected, it was very tender. He flinched but did not pull his foot away. I found the thyroid reflex very sensitive to pressure, as well as the adrenal and gonad reflexes. Also the reflex to the thymus was painful to the touch. I did not know exactly what this had to do with his condition, but there was definitely some connection there.

As I went over both feet gently, I found the reflexes on one foot more sensitive than the ones on the other. This seems to be general in cases of mental disorders.

I was unable to see if I had helped Mr. D. very much, but when I had completed a very short session, I suggested that he go to sleep now, and that I could come back to reflex his feet again in two days. His eyes watched me warily but he did not offer to move from his position.

I told Mrs. D. that I thought he would sleep if left alone, and because she looked so harassed I talked her into letting me give her a mini reflex workout before I left.

Mrs. D. telephoned me the next day to say that she lay down on the sofa after I left and had gone to sleep, and when she woke up and looked in on her husband, he was sleeping soundly.

When I went back in two days as I had promised, I found Mr. D. sitting on the edge of the bed with a sheet pulled over him. I could see a glimmer of recognition in his eyes as he stretched out his foot to me. I pulled up a chair, and he quickly put both feet in my lap. He had remembered, and at least subconsciously knew that he had been helped, and that this was Nature's way of releasing his built-up tensions and distraught emotions.

I worked the reflexes a little more severely this time since he didn't seem to mind. As I left, I told him I would return in two days.

To my surprise, on my third visit, I found both Mr. D. and Mrs. D. in the front room. Mr. D. was dressed and shaved.

"He still won't talk to me, or eat with me, but he keeps looking for someone. I'm sure it is you. I'm so thankful to you—I know you have saved his life," said Mrs. D.

"No, don't thank me," I said. "I only gave Nature a boost by stimulating the reflexes as they were meant to be stimulated in the first place. You could have done as much if you had understood about the reflexes and the technique of working them."

I suggested that we wait three days for the next treatment, and that we should see much improvement by then.

It was most gratifying to watch Mr. D.'s improvement after that, and he returned to teaching within six weeks.

I taught both Mr. and Mrs. D. how to keep the pituitary gland active and in good health by reflexing the center of the big toe on each foot. I warned them that if at any time it showed the least tenderness, it must be reflexed every other day or two until all tenderness left.

There are, of course, those whom we cannot treat with such satisfying results, but still reflexology can help to some extent and bring some semblance of relief.

A Case of Cerebral Palsy Helped

A boy was brought to my office so completely helpless that his mother had to carry him in from the car. He was 14 years of age, and had suffered from cerebral palsy from the time he was a baby. His body was terribly twisted, and he had no control over his arms, legs, or head. He had great difficulty in his speech but was able to say a few words with great effort.

When we put him in the chair the first time, he was very nervous and frightened, and asked if I was going to use an instrument. The boy had been to so many doctors and had been given so many shots and tests that he was frightened of everyone to whom his mother took him for treatment. She explained that there was just a chair for him to sit in, and one for me to sit on, and that there were no machines of any kind, but as she was not familiar with reflexology, she was unable to tell him what I was going to do.

When I lifted his feet into position for reflexing, I was shocked to see how twisted the poor things were. He seemed very frightened when I started to remove his shoes. I explained that I was going to rub his feet, and that some of the places would hurt but all he had to do was tell me and I would be very gentle. I didn't know until later that the boy was also blind.

Of course, both his mother and I knew that reflexology would not cure him, but neither did we know how much help it could bring him. Since he was very distressed, we hoped that it would at least be of some help in calming his nerves. As soon as he understood that I would merely reflex his feet, he relaxed and seemed to enjoy it.

His feet were so curled and misshapen that it was very difficult to work on them. In addition, they were in constant motion. There were no definite reflexes that I could work on except the toes and heel. However, I went over his feet the best I could, experimenting with the press-and-roll motion. In a case like this, we never know which reflex we might stimulate to give Nature's boost, thereby starting a chemical reaction of the whole system that could restore health to parts of the body that were not recognized as being the seat of the ailment.

In treating with reflexology, I have learned to expect surprises of all kinds. In this case, the hands needed reflexing also, as they were so deformed and crippled that he was unable to hold anything, let alone be handled enough to stimulate their reflexes.

In this particular case, we felt that we may have improved his hearing, and to some extent his mental capacities. The reflex sessions did help his nerves to a great extent, and also his disposition. My daughter, age 14 at the time, would come in after school and he showed an increasing interest in her and her chatter. He eventually developed into one of the happiest-natured children I ever knew. Occasionally, I would take other children to visit him.

How wonderful it would be if all those who are living restricted lives could be helped by reflexology, thus providing them with a happier existence!

OVERCOMING MENTAL DEPRESSION

Although it is possible to obtain relief from physical discomforts through the techniques of reflexology, body tensions can result from poor thinking habits. Everyone should assume a cheerful, optimistic attitude toward life's problems and develop spiritual strengths by taking positive steps to learn as much as possible about God's great love for all His people. No one is meant to live in fear and want, in poor health, or in a state of hopelessness. Reflexology can do much to change our desperate preoccupation with mental and physical discomforts without resorting to drugs or other escape routes.

A Case of Depression Healed

One day a man came to the office, complaining that he felt very depressed, couldn't find any interest in life any more, and sometimes felt like "ending it all" because he was a "burden" to his family and friends.

As a matter of fact, he was not a burden to his family, and had many fine friends. He worked hard and supplied his family with luxuries, was apparently in good health, and had no special worries. The man had everything in the world to be thankful for, and here he was, talking of ending his life!

After talking with him for awhile, I asked him to sit in the chair and remove his shoes and socks. The first reflex I look for is the one to the pituitary gland in the center of the big toe. It was very tender, and he nearly jumped out of the chair. "What did you do—stick a needle in my toe?" he asked.

I explained that I had merely used the edge of my thumb to press into his toe, and that the "needle" he thought he felt was already inside the toe. I showed him how to do it for himself, and he was amazed at the painful result. I told him this was probably the cause of his unhappiness, the little culprit that was the source of his mental depression and loss of interest in life. I mentioned further that the pituitary was the "king gland" in his body and acted as a kind of harmonizer of the whole system. Indeed, through a course of experiments made by an American medical doctor, it has been discovered that bullying, lying, vagrancy, and moroseness in children had been traced to a faulty pituitary gland.

Also, I explained that the reflex to the pineal gland, which was located in his big toe, was another clue, as it is an organizer of harmony in the other endocrine glands, and that the improper functioning of these glands could be normalized by working the reflexes located in the bottom of the feet. He was very interested in my method of reflex and asked me to proceed, no matter how painful it might be.

As I went over each reflex, I found the areas of the endocrine glands to be the most sensitive, but none was so tender as the one in the big toe. I kept returning to give it a few seconds of stimulation, and as I had learned to expect with anyone in his mental state, the reflexology was more tender in one foot than in the other.

My patient became very relaxed, and on leaving, he said, "You know, I think the world looks better to me already! How soon can I come back?"

This man needed only six reflex sessions in all to restore his will to live and acquire a renewed zest for life.

He was so grateful for his new lease on life that he asked me to give him lessons on reflexology techniques. Now he devotes a lot of his own time working the reflexes of all who ask him for help with health problems.

And that is why this book has been written . . . so that you, too, can give yourself, or anyone else, a natural secret which will improve circulation and promote renewed health and efficiency of all glands and organs.

In your hands, you now hold a new hope to freedom from pain and illness for all people. Here is a way to health naturally, without drugs or surgery . . . so learn it well, and use it to benefit others and make life healthier and happier for yourself!

Index

SELF-HELP REFLEXOLOGY TOOLS

Stirling Enterprises, Inc. distributes Mildred Carter's Reflexology Tools. If you are interested in obtaining any of the reflex tools shown in this book, simply call 1-800-766-3668, for a free catalog of natural health products.

> Stirling's order hours are Monday through Friday 9:00 A.M. to 3:00 P.M. Pacific Time.

Visit Mildred Carter Reflexology @ www.mcreflexology.com for express online ordering. Just select the items you want and order within minutes.

Remember, shopping by catalog or online for Reflexology products is fast, safe and easy. You can shop while comfortable, plus it saves you time and gas money looking for these unique and helpful products.

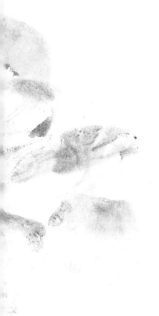